Tots About

The NCT Baby and Toddler Guide to Guildford

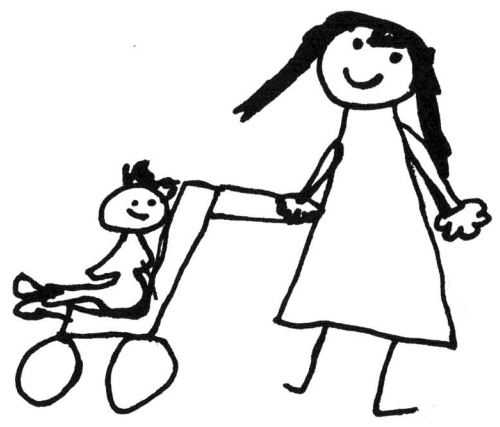

edited by Emma Tappenden

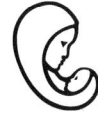

First published in 2002 by Guildford National Childbirth Trust.

This new revised edition published 2007.

Copyright © 2007, 2002 Guildford National Childbirth Trust.
c/o Alexandra House, Oldham Terrace, London, W3 6NH.
totsabouttown@nctguildford.org.uk
www.nctguildford.org.uk

The moral right of the authors has been asserted.

The views and opinions expressed in this
publication are not necessarily those of the National Childbirth Trust

All rights reserved.
No part of this publication may be reproduced,
stored in a retrieval system, or transmitted, in any form
or by any means, without the prior permission in writing of the publisher,
nor be otherwise circulated in any form of binding or cover other
than that in which it is published and without a similar
condition, including this condition being imposed
on the subsequent purchaser.

A CIP catalogue record for this book
is available from the British Library.

ISBN 978-0-9541840-1-8

Produced in association with the National Childbirth Trust.
Registered Office: Alexandra House, Oldham Terrace, London, W3 6NH.
www.nct.org.uk
Registered charity no: 801395
Registered company no: 2370573

The National Childbirth Trust wants all parents to have
an experience of pregnancy, birth and early parenthood that enriches
their lives and gives them confidence in being a parent.

Typeset by Debbie Beasley
Printed and bound in Great Britain
by Polestar Wheatons, Hennock Road, Marsh Barton, Exeter, Devon, EX2 8RP.

Contents

Introduction	1
1 All about the NCT	**3**
The National Childbirth Trust	3
Guildford NCT	5
2 Things to do	**11**
Parent/Carer and Toddler Groups	12
Sporting activities	22
Gymnastics	23
Trampolining	27
Football	28
Tennis	29
Ice Skating	29
Swimming	29
Soft Play	38
Music Groups	46
Signing	49
Cinema and Theatre	51
Baby Massage/Baby Yoga	54
Dance	58
Art Activities	57
Story Time	59
Ante/Postnatal Exercise	60
Holiday Activities	64
3 Places to Visit	**67**
Farms	68
Aquariums, Bird Parks and Zoos	71
Garden Centres	74
Duck Feeding and Paddling	77
National Trust (NT) Houses and Gardens	79
Parks and Gardens	83
Walks and Family Cycling Trips and Days Out	86
Theme Parks	92
Trains, Cars and Aeroplanes	97
Other Days Out	98
Seasonal Events – Spring	100
Seasonal Events – Summer	101
Seasonal Events – Autumn	102
Seasonal Events – Winter	104
Playgrounds	104
	106
4 Public Transport	**115**
Using public transport	116
Out and about with a pushchair…	117
…by bus	117
…by train	117
5 Shopping	**119**
Clothes	120
Shoes	123
Baby essentials and maternity wear	125
Toys and Books	128
General Shops	132
Online/Catalogues	133
Second Hand Bargains	137
Toilets and Changing Facilities	138

Contents

6 Eating Out — 140
Restaurants — 141
Cafés — 150
Pubs and Bars — 156
Takeaways — 161

7 Services — 166
Parties — 167
Venues — 167
Party Equipment Hire — 171
Party Accessories — 172
Entertainers — 174
Catering Equipment Hire — 174
Hairdressers — 175
Photographers — 178
Washable Nappies — 179
Eco-friendly disposables — 185
Other eco-friendly disposables — 186
Information Centres — 186

8 Health and Welfare — 190
Healthcare Provision – GP Surgeries — 191
Health Visitors — 192
Alternative therapies — 193
Finding a Dentist — 195
If Your Child Needs Glasses... — 196
Breastfeeding — 197

9 Childcare — 199
Daycare Nurseries — 200
Preschools — 201
Childminders — 202
Crèche — 203
Nannies — 204
Au pairs — 205
Mother's Help — 205
Babysitting — 206
Paying for it — 206
Nursery Education Grant — 206
Childcare Voucher Schemes — 207

Introduction

When I joined Guildford *NCT* in January 2004, one of the first things I did was buy *Tots about Town*, at a 'Starters Evening'. At the time I was told: 'It's a great book, but phone before you go along to activities as some of the times are out of date.'

I dipped in and out of the book over the next couple of months before my son William was born, and found the whole list of places that I'd never heard of before a bit daunting. However, within a couple of months of his birth in March, it became indispensable to me for looking up where to shop, eat, and change him, where to take him out, and for planning the things that we could do on the days that I didn't work (or work out which days to work around the things I wanted to do with him!) When I became chair in early 2005, we knew the book was out of date, but realising it was still valuable, we continued giving it away at nearly new sales and coffee mornings for a donation. During 2005 and 2006 at several committee meetings, it was mentioned that an update of the book was a project that needed 'doing', but everyone kept their hands firmly down when asked who wanted to get the ball rolling. Finally after a couple of false starts, I encouraged (or should that be, bullied) a team into meeting at my house to start the second edition of *Tots about Town*.

Having never even written a magazine article before, let alone a book, I had no idea what to do; so I just chaired the meetings, and shouted for help loudly and regularly until behold – a whole range of excellent, talented and knowledgeable assistance came along to produce this wonderful update of our favourite toddler guide.

This book is modelled very closely on the fantastic first edition that Jo Rew and her team produced so successfully in 2002 – we've even asked some of the original contributors to come back and give their updated take on things. The book is once again based on recommendations from over a hundred local parents for children up to the age of three. But having a three-year-old myself, I know from reading the reviews that there are another hundred activities to keep William occupied up to school age and beyond.

Introduction

All the opinions in this book are very personal, and one great thing that I have found, is that you can listen to all sides and then work out what you'd like to do, visit or take part in.

I hope you enjoy this updated version of *Tots about Town*, there are so many things for you and your family to enjoy in the Guildford area; it is a great place to bring up a family, and hopefully with this guide at your side, you will be able to make full use of all there is on offer over the coming weeks and months and years.

Claire Brown, mum of William

A note from the editor

If you wanted a book that gives even more recommendations of things to do and places to visit, and more advice on welfare and childcare, then this is the book for you. Such has been the enthusiasm from mums and dads in Guildford to have a new and revised version of *Tots About Town*, that we have a particularly wide content within this edition. Also, as the internet is now used so widely, we have included websites and email addresses where they exist. So, in an effort to keep the number of pages down a bit, and in the knowledge that people really only need the first line of an address and postcode in order to find a place, towns and counties have only been named where they are outside Guildford.

Please do note, that although we have taken great care to check that all contact details are current and correct, they are all subject to change as they can go out of date very quickly, especially with shops opening and closing every few weeks, and new groups starting up and old ones running their course. So do use the contact details provided, or look online, and check the maps included towards the end of the book, before you set out on an unknown expedition with babes and/or toddlers in tow!

Finally, I must point out that the advertisers in this book have been approached as they have already advertised with the *NCT* in Guildford, or have services or facilities that tie-in with the information we have provided. Having the advert in this book does not constitute its endorsement by the *NCT*, although all comply with the advertising standards and ethics that the *NCT* sets.

I'd also like to take this opportunity to personally thank Claire for handing me the reins on this project, and the *Tots About Town* committee for giving me the freedom and scope I needed to get this book published. It's been an extremely rewarding challenge! See also acknowledgements at the end of the book.

Emma Tappenden, mum of Charlotte and Louis

1
All about the NCT

Lise Faccinello, mum of Livi and Luca

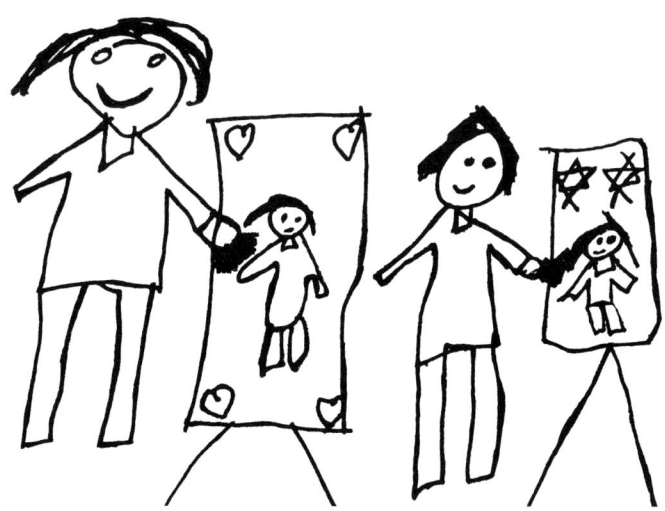

The National Childbirth Trust

Mention the *NCT* to some people and they recoil in horror, no doubt wondering how they never noticed that you were the *beanbags and lentils* type. What is it about the *National Childbirth Trust*? Others think it's called the *Natural* Childbirth Trust, and that becoming a member is tantamount to joining an evangelical sect; you will be forced to give birth in a field under a full moon chanting ancient pagan rites and, what is more, be granted no pain relief whatsoever in your moment of need. Others still, like myself, thought that you had to have a shopping account with *Fortnum and Masons* before your membership would be accepted. I was sure my battered little car would not pass muster with the wealthy members, or worse, it would be mown down, unseen from the heights of one of their capacious off-road runabouts. Well, my experience resembled none of the above, thank goodness. Here is what it was really like.

From the moment I saw the little blue line, I began to visualise life *after birth* with a combination of rose tinted anticipation and trepidation. I had just moved, and didn't know a soul where we lived. We had no family nearby,

All about the NCT

either. What would I do once my husband went back to work? Would I just have to stay in all day going bonkers? I was really worried about my impending isolation. It was my friend, Sue, who persuaded me that I would meet people through the NCT. She had an 18 month head start and had been through the same thing. She also told me how good the classes were. So, I went ahead and joined.

It was amazing how quickly we gelled in those classes. Everyone was going through the same experience, I suppose, making the transition from irresponsibility (in my case, at least) to parenthood. To cut a long story short, we all became friends, and got together regularly after our babies were born. There's probably nothing so bonding as swapping sleepless-night stories or new-parent anxieties with equally sleepless new friends. Sadly, we had to leave our old NCT crowd with our move to Guildford when Livi was five months old. It was quite a wrench, but we still keep in touch. The move to Guildford was very stressful and Livi started sleeping badly, so I really needed some friendly human contact. This is when the NCT became a real life-saver for me. I must have gone to every event in the newsletter when I first came here. I gradually got to know more and more people as time went by, and made some really good friends.

And going back to what I was saying earlier, I really don't think there's an NCT 'type'. On the contrary, the people I come across seem to be quite diverse. (They certainly don't all sit around swapping favourite lentil recipes, and my car, I am pleased to say, is still intact). In fact, the only thing you could say everyone in the NCT has in common is that they're all parents.

So it's pretty clear that the NCT provides a great support network for parents locally, but it also does important work on a national level. Pregnancy and early parenthood can be a vulnerable time, and the NCT acts as a powerful voice on antenatal, birth and postnatal issues, and works to improve the childbirth experience for everyone. It has successfully campaigned for the presence of partners at birth, and for a mother's right to have her baby close by her at the hospital. The NCT does not dictate to parents, but promotes the principle of informed choice for women and their partners. It is the largest and best known childbirth and parenting charity in Europe, with over 70,000 members across the UK.

As a charity, the NCT depends on subscriptions. In 2007 the fees for new members are £39.00 a year, and £29.00 for subsequent years. You can pay quarterly, and if you are on family credit or income support, the subscription is just £1.00. If you would like to know more about the NCT or its services, or would like to get in touch with your local branch, call (0870) 444 8707, or log onto the website at www.nct.org.uk. For support on breastfeeding, call (0870) 444 8708.

All about the NCT

Guildford NCT (http://nctguildford.org.uk)

We are an active branch, with over 350 members. Run by local parents for local parents, we provide a range of services, which are available to everyone. Here are some of the activities and social events going on. In the true style of this book people who have used the services have given us a comment, so you can hear about them from the horse's mouth.

Antenatal Classes

'I really recommend the *NCT*'s antenatal classes; we had an excellent teacher and the course complements the *Royal Surrey's* classes very well. It also gives you an instant introduction to a set of local people with babies the same age, so you are bound to find some friends.'
Victoria, mum of Catherine

Bra-fitting Service

'I found the bra-fitting service very helpful. I actually went to the bra fitter's house and it was much more pleasant being fitted in the comfort of someone's house than a shop with cramped changing facilities. The ranges of bras that the *NCT* stocked were also good and I was very pleased with the ones that I bought.'
Katherine, mum of Holly and Hazel

Breastfeeding Support

Breastfeeding does not always go smoothly in the beginning. Our breastfeeding counsellors offer support and information on any aspect of breastfeeding and will not question a mother's right to choose her own method of feeding her baby.

Breast Pumps

You can hire an electric breast pump from the branch. These are particularly useful for helping to breastfeed premature or sick babies.

Branch Library

We have a selection of books on a range of subjects, from pregnancy to parenting. You can see a complete list on our website at *www.nct.org.uk/branches/guildford*.

All about the NCT

'Bring and Share' Suppers

'Everyone brings along some food, which greatly lightens the burden of hosting, these evenings, which are a lovely opportunity to chat to familiar mums without any distractions from little ones and also to meet other mums in your area.'
Liz, mum of Thomas

Bumps and Babes

'These are coffee mornings and afternoon teas for pregnant parents and those with new babies – usually up to six months. They are an opportunity to meet up with others in the local area without lots of older babies and toddlers.'
Claire, mum of William

Coffee Mornings

'These are usually held in someone's house and are a great way for mums to catch up with each other while their little ones explore someone else's toys. They are especially good for new mums who want to meet others going through those difficult first few weeks or for those that are new to the area.'
Liz, mum of Thomas

Home Birth Contact

'Anyone thinking about having a home birth can ring a local mum, who's had two home births herself, for an informal chat. She will offer local, practical information and will try to answer any questions you have. (You can find her number in the newsletter.)'
Terri Walter, 'local mum' of Ben, Chloe and Philippa

Local Experience Register

The branch holds a register of local people who have experienced difficulties, and who can support others going through similar experiences. These range from problems during pregnancy to illness or the death of a child.

Maternity Services Liaison Committee (MSLC)

'The MSLC at the *Royal Surrey County Hospital* is an open forum between families and staff involved with maternity care. Its goal is to foster strong links between the

community and Health Authority for the continued improvement of the quality of maternity care. It is rewarding to be part of something that makes a real difference to the maternity care available locally. Meetings are held every two months and interesting projects often arise that can be readily fitted into life as a busy parent. Since joining the MSLC as an NCT representative I have become involved with the *Save the Royal Surrey Campaign* and a research project to gain feedback from mothers who have recently given birth at the hospital. New parents are always welcome to join.'
Beth (NCT representative at the Royal Surrey MSLC), mum of Abigail

National Experience Register

The National *NCT* holds a more extensive register covering a huge range of parents' experiences. Please call (0870) 4448707 for more information.

NCT Swimming
[See also main entry under Things to do]

'This is a lovely way to introduce your child to the water. The session runs on a Tuesday afternoon in the teaching pool at Guildford *Spectrum*. In addition to the usual lifeguards, a swimming instructor is also on hand, which means that you can take more than one child, and have a helping hand in and out of the pool with babes-in-arms. Arm-floats are available, and there are changing mats beside the pool. That way you can change your babies immediately before and after your swim so they don't get too cold. There are plenty of toys in the water, which encourages swimming as the child strives to reach them. Oh, and it's really cheap too – always a bonus! Family changing rooms are reasonable with baby changing pods and baby seats for while you change, although can be quite chilly.'
Emma, mum of Charlotte and Louis

Nearly New Sales
[All branch sales are listed on the main NCT website – www.nct.org.uk.]

'This is the place to get all of those baby and toddler bits that you would really like but don't want to pay for brand new. It is also the place to sell on items that junior has grown out of. You name it, you can find it, from baby cribs, baby baths, cots and stair-gates, to dressing up clothes, tricycles, jigsaws and *Duplo* etc. Virtually all of your child's wardrobe could be purchased at one sale. Also, if you need to advise Santa on where he can acquire the necessary items at low cost, tell him to keep watch in the branch newsletter for the dates, then turn up on the day.

There is a nominal charge for entry, and generally a queue has formed before the sale starts. If you want to shop early, get first pick and avoid the crowds, then volunteer to help on the day. Helpers generally do a three to four hour shift before, during or after the sale. If you would like to volunteer, check in the newsletter for the person to contact.'
Maggie, mum of Alice and Katy

'Sales run three times a year: spring for clothing, equipment and toys; autumn for clothing and equipment sale; followed a month later by the toy sale. Fabulous opportunity for the first-time mum to pick up pretty much everything she needs for her new baby at a fraction of the cost of buying new.'
Sonya, mum of Eleanor and Charles

Newsletter

'Over the last couple of years we have gone 'back to basics' on the main parenting themes that each newsletter focuses on. We try to have broad topics that will be relevant to everyone, but also show different personal perspectives. We have boosted our breastfeeding pages to give nursing mothers even more guidance and support, and we also now have 'food pages', which reveal nutritional know-how and fabulous recipe ideas for pregnancy, babies and families. The newsletter comprises the themed articles along with *NCT* branch and national news, positions vacant, volunteering opportunities, experience registers, and upcoming events, such as local coffee mornings and informal get-togethers. Many readers even find the adverts useful in seeking goods and services for their families. The newsletter is published quarterly and contains useful numbers/contact details you might need at different points in your parenting career. We always welcome submissions from mums, dads, health professionals and anyone else who'd like to share their views.'
Paige Sinkler, newsletter editor and mum of Miranda and Leo

New To ... Meals

'Guildford *NCT* runs regular monthly evenings aimed at getting together those that are new to having a baby, new to the area, or new to the *NCT*. This is often the first event that couples come to when they start with the *NCT*. The evenings are alternately a social shared supper, and a talk about subjects relevant to pregnant or new parents, such as nutrition; environmental issues including nappies; baby kits and gadgets; and exercise.'
Claire, mum of William

One-Off Events

We really are a busy bunch! On top of all of the events in our regular diary, we also organise one-off events quite regularly, like dances, or a 'no-bang' firework display that aims not to scare babies and toddlers.

Postnatal Classes (Early Days Classes)

Groups of mums (and/or dads) of babies under six months old are put together with others with babies of a similar age. They take place during the day and you bring your baby along.

'Format is a different topic each week. Classes run by a very knowledgeable postnatal teacher. Very informative and give you lots of practical information. Discussion groups enable you to compare notes and experiences with other mums of babies of a similar age. It is so valuable to talk to others going through exactly the same things as you and realise you are not alone.'
Helen, mum of Dominic and Laura

'Postnatal courses are aimed at mothers (or fathers) with babies under six months of age and take place during the day with meetings being held weekly over a period of six weeks. Parents attend with their babies. Run by a trained and accredited group leader, *Early Days* courses give the opportunity to discuss your thoughts, concerns and needs about being a new parent. By sharing ideas and experiences and helping others to do the same, parents can support each other and learn more about their skills as parents. These courses explore a range of approaches to important parenting issues so that you have the confidence to make the right decisions for your baby. Group leaders won't give 'talks' about child development and first aid, but they will have up-to-date information to help you decide what is best for your baby, you and your family.'
Catherine Wands, postnatal student and mum of Elisabeth, William and Emma

Refresher Classes

'Having fallen pregnant with my second child it was suggested that I attend a refresher class. I was a little sceptical as surely I knew it all from the first time around just two years prior? Terri led the class; she is clearly very experienced so I felt in good hands. Her 'classroom' is set within her home and is really comfortable; she even supplied birthing balls for us to perch on and I met up with five other mums (only one of which I knew). I found the classes to be really informative, theoretical and practical. We had plenty

All about the NCT

of opportunity to share about our first experiences and felt empowered to take on the second arrival. We also had a lot of laughs and I made some super new friends – I am so very pleased I did attend.'
Vicki, mum of George and Finlay

Valley Cushion Hire

A valley cushion is specially designed to relieve pressure on stitches, tears, bruising and haemorrhoids before or after birth.

Volunteering

'I've enjoyed being an *NCT* volunteer and got a great deal out of it. As lots of people are needed in order to spread the work, it's easy – and much valued – to join in with something simple. I started delivering a few newsletters to my local streets (no hardship as I was pacing those streets with my baby in the pram anyway) and then got more involved once my daughter was a bit older.'
Victoria, mum of Catherine

For further information on local *NCT* services or events, please call us on:

Membership	0870 4609633
Class Bookings	0870 4609632
Nearly New Sales	0870 4609641
General Enquiries	0870 4609631

2
Things to Do

Helen Ayscough, mum of Dominic and Laura
Lynn Egan, mum of Ella

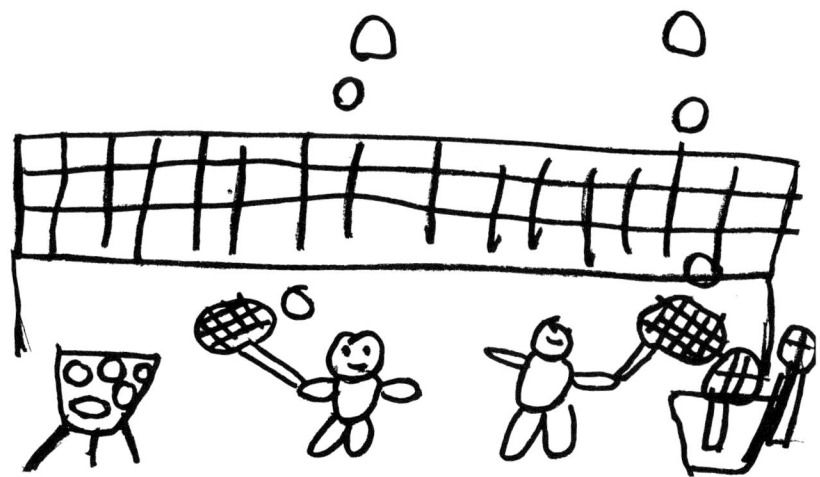

After compiling this section, we now believe that if there was a national survey of top ten places to live for things to do with under-fives, Guildford and surrounds must be near the top of the list. All the carer needs is enough energy to keep up with the kids. For a start, there are nearly forty playgroups listed; you could fill your week with those alone! OK, no need to visit all of them, but seriously please do try one or two at least, they are a great way for both the carer and baby to enter into the wider social world.

Our tour of *'Things to Do'* continues with sporting activities. These are usually more structured activities, but great for building confidence and burning off energy. We then have swimming recommendations for both lessons and informal opportunities to splash about. Soft play areas are a 'must-visit', and we have a comprehensive set of reviews to help you make an informed choice of where to go. We then move on to more relaxing things to do such as music groups, sing and sign, and cinema and theatre. If you fancy a little chill out time with your baby, read through the reviews written about baby massage and baby yoga. For all those budding artists, the section reviewing art activities

Things to Do

gives ideas and suggestions on where you can go for little people to have fun with a paintbrush. If after all of this you have enough energy and fancy burning some more, the next section details where you can go to fitness classes with or without your baby. This chapter then closes with a review of things to do during holidays when some of your usual activities may not be running. So, sit back, grab a cuppa and happy reading.

Parent/Carer and Toddler Groups

These groups are a must at some point for any carer of 0 to five-year-olds. They are a vital lifeline for first-time mums, a place to bring baby, get out of the house, have a chat and a coffee with other first-time mums in the same boat. One first-time mum, who pre-baby vowed never to step foot into one, now says how great her local group is. She has found a childminder for her child there and made many new friends.

For toddlers on the move, they provide a huge variety of toys, activities and other children to keep the little ones occupied. They are a good place to use as a venue to carry on meeting with your postnatal group, and if you continue there's a good chance that you'll make lots of other long-term friends there. Often carers end up loyal to one or two groups that fit the best into their weekly routine.

What exactly is a 'parent and toddler group'? These groups are open to anyone who is a carer, not just mum or dad – grandparents, guardian, nanny, childminder, au pair or any adult with babies or toddlers in their care. All the baby and toddler groups in Guildford or surrounds have facilities for preschool children aged 0 to five. The groups are generally run by volunteers, most run only in term-time, but any exceptions are noted at the end of this chapter in the *'Holiday Activities'* section. Most have a small entrance fee, some have a waiting list system, but the majority allow you to turn up as and when you desire. Each group operates differently – all have a selection of toys; some have craft activities; often there is a song and/or story time at the end. There is always plenty of time for free play.

Parent and toddler groups are not registered with the local authority and therefore children remain the responsibility of the parent/carer at all times during the session. The pages that follow list as many toddler groups in the Guildford and surrounding area as we could find. Times of groups do change occasionally, so if you are planning a visit to a new toddler group you should probably ring first to confirm details.

Finally, please do not be upset if there are no comments included about your local group – this has no bearing on the individual merit of your group. We have included comments where we have received them. Just go along and try the groups out for yourself. Enjoy!

Quick Reference Guide to toddler groups
(Cen) = Central, NW = Northwest, E = East, V = Villages

Monday	AM – St Joseph's Church Toddler Group (Cen) – Teddies & Co (NW)	PM – Jacobs Well Toddler Group (E) – New Horizons Toddler Group (NW)
Tuesday	AM – Getaway Club (Cen) – Guildford Children's Centre Play & Learn (Cen) – Stoke Toddler Group (Cen) – Teddy Bear Club (Cen) – Manor Road Toddler Group (NW) – St Francis Baby & Toddler Group (NW) – St Pius Toddler Group (E) – Little Lambs Playgroup (E) – Chilworth Toddler Group (V)	PM – Guildford Children's Centre Play & Learn (NW) – Tuesday Club (E) – Active Tots (E)
Wednesday	AM – Tiny Treasures (Cen) – St Nicolas Baby & Toddler Group (Cen) – Adults, Babies and Children (ABC) (E) – Evangelical Church Group (E) – Shalford Baby and Toddler Group (V) – Bramley Toddler Group (V)	PM – Burpham Church of the Holy Spirit (E)
Thursday	AM – St. Saviour's Baby & Toddler Groups (Cen) – Guildford United Reformed Church (Cen) – C.A.M.E.O (NW) – St Albans Parent & Toddler Group (NW)	PM – Teddies & Co (NW) – Guildford Children's Centre Play & Learn (NW) – St John's Mother & Toddler Group (E) – Koala Club (V)
Friday	AM – All Saints Church Toddler Group (Cen) – Millmead Baptist Church Centre (Cen) – Little Lambs Playgroup (E) – Caterpillar Café (E) – Guildford Twins Club (E)	PM – Guildford Children's Centre Play & Learn (Cen)

Things to Do

Central Guildford

All Saints Church Mother and Toddler Group
Vicarage Gate
Onslow Village
GU2 7QJ
(01483) 576511 (Liz Robinson)
(01483) 533979 (Claire Austen)
information@allsaintschurchgfd.org.uk
www.allsaintschurchgfd.org.uk
Friday 9.30 – 11.00 am

'Edward was just fascinated by the number of people there – it was very busy!! Lots of mums from Onslow Village bring their children along so it is a good opportunity to meet people and there are themes to some sessions. Towards the end of the session, there is a 'singalong' while the toys are put away. It costs £1.00 (which includes a drink and a biscuit!) There are play mats and large toys for younger ones as well as other toys for the older children.'
Katy, mum of Edward

Getaway Club
Methodist Church Hall
Woodbridge Road (entrance side door on Wharf Road)
GU1 4RG
(01483) 571615 (Susan Snashall)
gmc.info@hotmail.com
www.guildfordmethodist.org
Term-time: Tuesday 10.00 – 11.30 am

'This is a smallish and friendly toddler group, which we enjoy. It takes place in a hall with lots of toys and ride-ons, a baby area and a different craft activity each week. There is a break halfway through for a drink, biscuit and a story, and then at the end there is singing.'
Tessa, mum of Daisy, Zach and Jake

Guildford Children's Centre (Town Centre site) – Play and Learn
York Road
GU1 4DU
(01483) 561652
info@guildfordchildrenscentre.surrey.sch.uk
www.guildfordchildrenscentre.surrey.sch.uk
Term-time: Friday 12.45 – 2.15 pm – for toddlers aged three and under
Term-time: Tuesday 9.15 – 11.00 am – for babies who are not yet walking

- The *Children's Centres* are state-run '*Early Excellence Centres*', funded by *SureStart* and *Surrey County Council*
- *Play and Learn* sessions for children under three, are allocated on a waiting list basis for other weekdays

[See also North Guildford site details under Northwest Guildford area p18]

'*Play and Learn* sessions are run by professional childcare staff, and the centre has great facilities. There are loads of toys, sand and water play, usually a craft activity such as painting or play dough, and outdoor play. Messy play is promoted, so don't wear your best clothes. It's a fantastic resource in the town centre. A donation of 50p is requested. You can help yourself to tea or coffee, and juice and fruit are offered to the children.'
Helen, mum of Dominic and Laura

Things to Do

Guildford United Reformed Church
Portsmouth Road
GU2 4BS
(01483) 536779 (Caroline Andrews)
(01483) 577532 (Jackie Sherwin)
(07794) 348745 (church)
admin@guildfordurc.org.uk
www.guildfordurc.org.uk
Term-time: Thursday 9.30 – 11.30 am

Millmead Baptist Church Centre
Millmead Centre
Bury Fields
GU2 4AZ
(01483) 575008 (Church)
(01483) 834533 (Karen Case-Green)
office@guildfordbaptist.org
www.guildfordbaptist.org
Friday 10.00 – 11.30 am
[Millmead operates a waiting list system, but you can just turn up for an initial trial session]

'The things I particularly like about Millmead are that during drink and snack time the staff read a story to the children in the quiet room, and in another room there are really good art activities in addition to the main hall filled with the usual toys and games. I like the fact there is some structure to the session. It's more than free-play alone. There is also nice cake for the grown-ups! The staff also arrange nice activities for mums called 'More than a Mum night' where mums get picked up and taken for a meal for a minimal cost.'
Kelly, mum of Albie and Poppy

St Joseph's Church Hall Mother and Toddler Group
York Road
Address for contact: St Joseph's Church
12 Eastgate Gardens
GU1 4AZ
(01483) 562704 (parish office)
(01483) 845012 (Leigh Ann Van Graan)
admin@stjo-guildford.co.uk
Term-time: Monday 10.00 – 11.30 am

'Large hall and fantastic selection of toys to keep youngsters amused, including ride-on toys and baby area. There is a play dough or craft table, plus jigsaws etc. A drink and fruit or biscuit are provided for children, and later a coffee or tea and bicky for mum/carer. It is rounded up with song time at the end – 'Sleeping Bunnies' is our favourite. There is always somebody friendly to talk to. When you first go, pick up a leaflet with session dates, as occasionally the group is not on during term-time when the hall is used for exams. This happens four or five times a year. The nearest car parks are Civic Hall or York Road.'
Helen, mum of Dominic and Laura

St Nicolas Baby and Toddler Group
1 Bury Street
GU2 4AW
(01483) 564526
parishoffice@stnicolas-guildford.fsnet.co.uk
Wednesday 9.30 – 11.30 am

'A friendly group in a nice bright hall. Most weeks there is a craft activity as well as tables laid out with jigsaws and play dough, and bigger toys on the floor. There

is tea and coffee for the mums and a drink and a biscuit for the kids. It's a popular group with a lot of regulars, but not as busy as some playgroups we've tried – which is great as the din doesn't get so loud that you can't have a chat, and if your little ones are new to playgroups, it's not overwhelming.'
Jo, mum of Stanley

St Saviour's Baby and Toddler Groups
Woodbridge Road
GU1 4QD
(01483) 455333
office@st-saviours.org.uk
www.st-saviours.org.uk
Term-time: Thursday 10.00 – 11.30 am [baby group sometimes additionally operates in holidays – call to check]

'There are three separate areas for babies and toddlers. Each section has lots of well-maintained, age-appropriate toys. The downstairs group is for babies, with a separate room to park prams and change nappies. There is one large room, half for tiny babies and the other half for those crawling or just starting to walk. Tea, coffee and biscuits are provided. For the toddler group, you park pushchairs in the church and go upstairs to a large area with big toys, ride-ons, dressing up, puzzles etc., and a separate craft area in the back for older children. Tea, coffee, squash and biscuits are provided for mums and kids. The cost is £1.00. The upstairs group is more structured, with snack time halfway through, and tidying up and singing at the end. It is a safe, friendly place that Audrey loves and it's great to get out and talk to other mums.'
Kelley, mum of Audrey

'This group is always popular. It is divided into a baby and small toddler area downstairs, and a separate older toddler group (equally popular) upstairs. Tea, coffee and biscuits are on offer, and volunteers are always welcoming. Changing facilities are available.'
Heather, mum of Jessica

Stoke Toddler Group
St John's Church
Stoke Road
GU1 1HB
(01483) 830457
www.stokechurch.org.uk
Tuesday 10.00 – 11.30 am

'This group is really easy to find, next to the Lido and Guildford College. There is always a very friendly atmosphere and the children have lots of fun running around in the hall, riding trikes, sliding down the slide, playing with cars and trains or sitting quietly in the reading corner. There is a craft table each week with sticking, painting, making cards etc. There is also a baby area with play gyms, toys and bouncy chairs. At the end we all move into a smaller room for a sing along, which the children love, especially 'Sleeping Bunnies', always a firm favourite!! I have found it a great toddler group for my boys. I can easily watch my eldest (20 months) while I am in the baby

area with his younger brother. Tea, coffee and biscuits are served too.'
Nicki, mum of Luke and Oliver

Teddy Bear Club
Guildford Park Church
Guildford Park Road
GU2 7NF
(01483) 575547
www.gpchurch.org.uk
Term-time: Tuesday 10.00 – 11.30 am
[Note: in addition to the toddler group the staff provide some fun evenings for mums at just a minimal cost]

'There's a long waiting list for a place here (we waited a year!) but because of this, once people have a place they tend to go regularly so it's very friendly and you get to know people well. Each week there's free play (with play dough, sand, ride-on toys, puzzles etc.) a bible story and song time with drinks and biscuits, and then the option of doing a craft activity and/or more free play. It's run by a really friendly and enthusiastic team and is definitely one of the most popular toddler groups in town.'
Jo, mum of James and Daisy

'Long waiting list, but worth the wait. It took Ella about nine months to get a place. The volunteers are always very friendly and helpful and it is a great way to meet other local mums and children. The set up is very clean and efficient. There are plenty of toys and activities. Tea and biscuits are included.'
Leena, mum of Ella

Tiny Treasures
Chertsey Street Baptist Church
Chertsey Street
GU1 4HL
(01483) 300238
www.chertseystreet.org.uk
Term-time: Wednesday 10.00 – 11.30 am

'I have been going here regularly for four years now. It never feels overcrowded. The rear hall is devoted to ride-ons initially, then converts into an area for tea/coffee, fruit and healthy snacks. There is a regular craft activity. The church itself is subdivided into dressing up, painting, play dough, trains, cars, and there is an enclosed area for infants and small babies. At the end there is a singing time and on alternate weeks a short bible story. There are always plenty of volunteers from the church on hand to help out, perhaps to hold your baby while you have a cup of tea or help your toddler with the craft.'
Alison, mum of Laura and Daniel

'We love this playgroup. Freyja (now four) has been going since she was a baby. The helpers are very friendly and ensure that new mums and children feel welcome. There are many nationalities attending this playgroup making it ideal for those who don't have family locally. The premises are large, with a play area and activities in a big hall as well as a separate room where refreshments are served. There are crafts and activities and the session ends with a story and singing.'
Thora, mum of Freyja

Things to Do

Northwest Guildford

C.A.M.E.O (for overseas students)
Emmanuel Church Hall
Stoughton
GU2 9SJ
(01483) 561603 (Church Office)
(01483) 872342 (Sue Handscombe)
www.emmanuelchurch.co.uk
2nd/4th Thursdays 10.45 am – 12.15 pm

Guildford Children's Centre (North Guildford site) – Play and Learn
Hazel Avenue
GU1 1NR
(01483) 566589
admin@guildfordchildrenscentre.surrey.sch.uk
www.guildfordchildrenscentre.surrey.sch.uk
Tuesday and Thursday 12.45 – 2.15 pm
[Additional sessions run during school holidays, see p64]

- The *Children's Centres* are state run '*Early Excellence Centres*', funded by *SureStart* and *Surrey County Council*
- In addition: *Play and Learn* sessions, for children under three, are allocated on a waiting list basis for other week days; ring for details

[See also town centre site details under Central Guildford p14]

'This is a large part of my children's social life – fantastic. Painting, soft play, sand play, gardens, water play, home corner, sticking, fruit, juice, tea, coffee and all for a small donation of 50p!! Brilliant. The town centre site also provides a special baby session on Tuesday mornings for non-crawlers [see page 14]. The *Children's Centre* provides *Play and Learn* sessions, day care nurseries and a preschool for three to five-year-olds, and also runs courses for parents in computing, English etc. There is a health visitor drop-in session on Mondays and also a postnatal support group among other things.'
Lisa, mum of Lewis, Scarlett, Dylan, Saffron, Jude, and Reuben

Manor Road Parent/Toddler Group
132 Manor Road
Stoughton
GU2 9NR
(01483) 571427(Fiona)
www.manorroadhall.org.uk
Tuesday 9.15 – 10.45 am

New Horizons Toddler Group
St Peters Church Hall
37 Hazel Avenue
Bellfields
(01483) 572078
www.stpetersguildford.org
Monday 1.45 – 3.00 pm

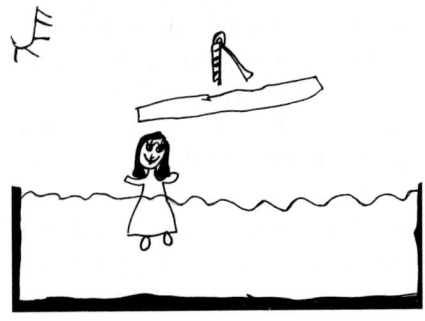

Things to Do

St Albans Parent & Toddler Group
St Albans Church Hall
Oak Hill
Wood Street Village
GU3 3ES
(01483) 233091 (Parish Office)
www.worplesdonparish.com
Thursday 9.45 – 11.15 am

St Francis Baby and Toddler Group
Beckingham Road
Stoughton
GU2 8JW
(01483) 504228 (Vicarage)
Tuesday 9.30 – 11.00 am

Teddies & Co Parent and Toddler Group
Emmanuel Church Hall
Shepherds Lane
Stoughton
GU2 9SJ
(01483) 561603 (Church Office)
(01483) 237766 (Sarah King re Mon)
(01483) 821835 (Sylvia Levick re Thurs)
www.emmanuelchurch.co.uk
Monday 10.00 – 11.30 am (NOT 2nd Mondays); Thursday 1.00 – 2.30 pm

'I go to the Thursday group and it's very friendly, with a good selection of toys. You can take babies from a very young age because there is a small area that is protected away from the older ones. There are craft areas in the side rooms for older children to do supervised artwork, and tables are laid out in different parts of the main room with jigsaws and other activities. There is a break midway through where everyone has a drink with a story and songs. It's a great atmosphere, well structured and welcoming.'
Charlotte, mum of Karina

East Guildford

Adults, Babies and Children (ABC): Christchurch Parent and Toddler Group
Christ Church Hall
23 Waterden Road
GU1 2AZ
(01483) 567072 (Sarah Goodchild)
wwwChristchurchguildford.com
Term-time: Wednesday 9.30 – 11.30 am

'Very welcoming and thriving group with climbing frames, mini trampoline, ride-on toys, small craft table, baby area, etc. An active Christian offshoot group for anyone interested. Pull down changing table in the loo and sturdy step unit up to the basin for toddlers to wash their hands.'
Sonya, mum of Eleanor and Charles

'ABC is a welcoming and lively toddler group. The refreshments are great, with a choice of coffees and various types of tea, biscuits and healthy snacks and drinks for toddlers (there is a requested donation to cover costs).

The selection of toys is excellent with a good rotation of active toys including ride-ons, a climbing frame with slide, a mini trampoline, and quiet toys including a brio track, cars and garage and a home corner. Babies are provided

Things to Do

for on a carpeted area with toys and baby bouncers. There is usually a craft every other week to make and take home. The morning is rounded off by a singing and story time on the carpet area, and usually closes with an enthusiastic rendition of the *Hokey Cokey*! A really good place to make friends.'
Julie, mum of Eliot and Oliver

Caterpillar Café
Church of the Holy Spirit
New Inn Lane
Burpham
GU4 7HW
01483 571686 (Katie Thomas)
me@katiethomas.co.uk
www.burphamchurch.org.uk
Friday 10.00 – 11.30 am
[See also 'Holiday Activities' p64]

'This is a church-based toddler group. All preschool aged children are welcome, with their carers, to join us for a relaxed, friendly and informal morning of coffee and play. Older brothers and sisters are welcome during the holidays and on special occasions. As well as the usual toys we have separate areas for dressing up, puzzles and craft. We finish each session with singing.'
Sam, mum of Freya

Evangelical Church Group
Ockham Road North
East Horsley
KT24 6NU
www.horsleyec.org.uk
Wednesday 10.00 – 11.45 am

'Very nice welcome from the minister's wife Ann; lovely friendly group with lots of toys, some outside play as well, and crafts including painting and play dough. Lovely cup of tea with biccies and drinks for children too. Finishes with song time, lots of friendly helpers. Small contribution to attend.'
Vicki, mum of George and Finlay

Guildford Twins Club
Merrow Village Hall
Merrow
(01483) 825950 (Karen Mears)
rmears@ntlworld.com
www.tamba.org.uk/clubs.php
$2^{nd}/4^{th}$ Friday monthly 10.00 – 11.30 am

[Bi-monthly playgroup for parents/carers of twins and multiples; expectant mothers welcome. Does not run during Christmas and school summer holidays, but during others please ring to check.]

Jacobs Well Toddler Group
Village Hall
Jacobs Well Road
GU4 7PD
(01483) 560467 (Jacquie)
Monday 1.30 – 3.00 pm

Little Lambs Playgroup
Send Evangelical Church
Broadmead Road
Send
GU23 7AD
tots@sendec.org (Debbie Hurdle)
www.sendec.org
Tuesday and Friday 10.00 – 11.30 am

'A popular very well organised playgroup with a waiting list (we waited six months to get in.) Children have to leave at the end of the term they turn three. There is always a supervised craft table with art and puzzles, another with play dough, and once a term the paint comes out. There is a kitchen corner made up like a wendy house with plywood walls. There is also a small slide, plenty of prams and ride-on toys, and a separate babies' area. The session finishes with song time. Coffee is available for mums, and juice or water and biscuits or tooth-friendly breadsticks for kids. There are enough helpers that I have rarely struggled being there with two kids 15 months apart in age. I shall be very sad when Alice turns three next term and will no longer be eligible to go.'
Maggie, mum of Alice and Katy

St John's Mother and Toddler Group
St John's community centre (next to St John's Church)
Trodds Lane
Merrow
(01483) 562609 (Alex)
(01483) 578884 (Sam)
Term-time: Thursday 2.00 – 3.30 pm

'A small but friendly playgroup. Lots of equipment and toys for babies and young toddlers and plenty of space to play in. Tea, squash and biscuits are provided, and there is a jolly singing session at the end.'
Claire, mum of Leni and Lottie

St Pius Toddler Group
St Pius Roman Catholic Church Hall
Lauston Close (off Horseshoe Lane East)
Merrow
GU1 2TS
(01483) 459097
Term-time: Tuesday 10.00 – 11.30 am

'A very friendly and welcoming playgroup with a lot to offer. In addition to a wide variety of toys, craft activities and play dough are available for older children. There is a separate area for babies and a good selection of baby toys. At break time squash, fruit and biscuits are available for children, and coffee and very nice biscuits for carers! The playgroup ends with a singing session including lots of action songs.'
Claire, mum of Leni and Lottie

'With weekly crafts, ride-ons, mini trampoline, and armchairs for mum to relax round the baby area.'
Sonya, mum of Eleanor and Charles

Tuesday Club
Merrow Methodist Church
Bushy Hill Drive
Merrow
GU4 7XR
(01483) 537655 (church)
(01483) 823498 (Jen Walker)
Term-time: Tuesday 1.45 – 2.15 pm

'This group is run by the very friendly ladies (and one man) from the church. There's a separate area for children to go charging around on ride-ons etc. and

Things to Do

there are tables set up with different activities e.g. cutting and sticking, play dough etc. There is a separate baby area.

In the summer when it's good weather the staff open up the enclosed garden at the back and have additional outdoor toys.'

Sally, mum of James

Surrounding Villages

Bramley Toddler Group
Holy Trinity Hall
Bramley
(01483) 898037 (Fran Lane)
Term-time: Wednesday 10.00 – 11.30 am

Chilworth Toddler Group
Village Hall
Chilworth
GU4 8LX
(01483) 570887 (Dawn Johnstone)
Tuesday 9.30 – 11.30 am

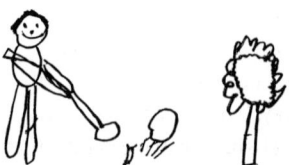

Koala Club Mother and Toddler Group
Bramley Village Hall
Hall Lane
Bramley
GU5 0AX
(01483) 892570 (Lisa)
Thursday 3.00 – 4.30 pm

Shalford Baby and Toddler Group
Methodist Hall
Kings Road
Shalford
GU4 8JU
(01483) 456920 (Kerry Darcy)
Term-time: Wednesday 10.00 – 11.30 am

'Ours is a very informal group. Ladies from the local church provide teas and coffees, while the children play. Then there is an informal singing session for the children at the end.'

Kerry, mum of Risa, Ayla and Lana

Sporting Activities

The variety of activities available for children in Guildford is amazing! Gym and other sports clubs are great for teaching motor skills, building confidence and for burning off loads of energy. Some clubs have a minimum age requirement and may have a waiting list, so please use the contact information below if necessary. Most of the clubs/classes listed below operate during term-time only, require booking, and usually require payment in advance, either termly of half-termly. Many though do offer a trial class.

Guildford *Spectrum* plays host to many activities mentioned throughout this section. It offers a little-known 'Cosmic Kids Club' scheme whereby you can earn discounts for various activities:

Cosmic Kids Club

[for three to ten-year-olds offering discounted rates on kids activities]
Guildford Spectrum Leisure Complex
Parkway
GU1 1UP
(01483) 443322
www.guildfordspectrum.co.uk

'Dominic got his 'Cosmic Kids Card' and 'Active Card' from the *Spectrum*. The main benefit for us is £1.00 off 'Specky's Pirates' soft play entry, we go there a lot! Other benefits include discounts off junior skate, leisure pool swim (off-peak times), tenpin bowling, basketball club and tennis club. Dominic also receives a regular newsletter. Sign up as a member (no membership fee applies) at the customer services office at the *Spectrum* (same floor as reception).'
Helen, mum of Dominic and Laura

Gymnastics

1 to 6 Gym Club

Mobile club, classes held at:
Merrow Club and Village Hall – Tues am
Merrow LA Fitness – Thurs pm
West Horsley Village Hall – Mon pm and Wed am
Ramster Gardens – Thurs am
(01483) 284744

'I have been a regular at *1 to 6 Gym Club* for four years since my daughter was nearly one, and since my son followed in her trainer-clad footprints two years later. The focus is on having fun and enjoying exercising while developing some physical confidence. There is a good range of activities to try with trampolines, balance beams, footballs and a large, padded tower to knock over at the end of the class. Great for burning off some energy. Mark, who runs the club, is wonderful with children of all ages. He really helped my daughter come out of her shell and develop some self-confidence. As well as gymnastics, they also play games like 'Musical statues' and 'Duck, Duck, Goose' which she particularly loved. My son gets plenty of football practice and looks forward to the classes so much he is having his third Birthday as a 'Gym Club' party. I highly recommend *1 to 6 Gym Club* and will be taking my third child when she is old enough to bounce on the trampoline.'
Lucy, mum of Abby, Henry and Alice

Gymnastics Factory

Pew Corner
Old Portsmouth Road
Guildford
GU3 1LP
(01483) 455060
info@gymnasticsfactory.co.uk
www.gymnasticsfactory.co.uk
[Classes run all day Monday to Saturday. Times vary according to age. Visit website for prices and timetables. See also 'Holiday Activities' p65 and 'Parties' p169]

'These gymnastics classes are absolutely fantastic! They run from age four months until adulthood. We are so glad we found them as I really wanted my son to get

Things to Do

active. These teacher-driven classes are the best we have come across. However, before you go there, you need to find out whether there is a space available in your desired class.'
Nadine, mum of Noah and Luca

Leatherhead & Dorking Gymnastics Club
Separate building adjacent to Leatherhead Leisure Centre car park
*Guildford Road
Fetcham
Leatherhead
KT22 9BL
(01372) 377718
www.leatherhead-gymnastics.org.uk*
[Website under construction at time of publication. Daily drop-in sessions 12.00 – 3.45 pm, from crawling to five years old; Structured classes from 18 months to 16 years; parent-free classes from age three. See also 'Holiday Activities' p66]

'This gymnastics club provides gymnastics classes, but also offers unsupervised drop-in sessions several times a day, during which children can use the gym equipment (including topless bouncy castle, foam pit, bars, etc) under the supervision of a parent or carer. It is open during the summer holidays too, which is great. It's small, but cheap and cheerful, as well as the fact it runs frequently!'
Paige, mum of Miranda and Leo

Rushmoor Gym
*The Gymnastics Centre
Pool Road
Aldershot
GU11 3SN
01252 320888
info@rushgym.co.uk (Colin and Bernie Wright)
www.rushgym.co.uk*
Term-time Playgym 9.30 – 10.30 am and 1.30 – 2.30 pm; £1.00 per person
Also holiday Playgym, see website for details. Also see under 'Soft Play' p43 and 'Holiday Activities' p66]

'Rushmoor runs '*Playgym*' sessions for an hour every day at 9.30 am and 1.30 pm. The gym is open to all parents and under-fives to go along and play in the gym. This club trains champions so is a very large, fully equipped gymnasium. Everything is very soft and padded, and quite often the floor is sprung underneath. For the toddlers there are soft play items placed on the floor area and a bouncy castle. The trampoline is at ground level. There is a strict rule that there is only one child on the trampoline at a time unless a coach is present, but this is not always adhered to. So kids get to balance on the beams, swing on the bars, run up and down the

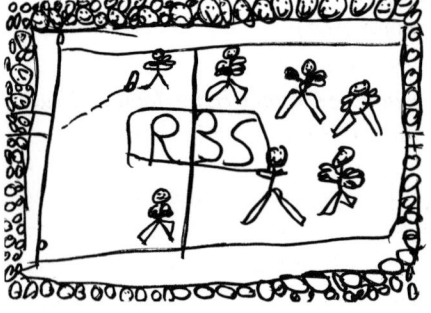

Things to Do

vault run and jump in the foam pit. It's an excellent way for them to burn off energy, and keeps you on your toes as you have to keep up with them! There is also a 'beginners' class for under-fives.
Emma, mum of Charlotte and Louis

Specky's Gympups
Guildford Spectrum
Leisure Complex
Parkway
GU1 1UP
(01483) 443322
www.guildfordspectrum.co.uk
Term-time: Tuesday pm and Thursday am classes.
[Times vary according to age. See website for details – type 'gympups' into search. See also 'Holiday Activities' p65]

'Gym classes from the age of 18 months upwards held in the sports arena at *Spectrum Leisure Complex*. There are large mats laid down on the floor for the entire Gympups area with proper gym equipment and large trampoline. There is a Gympups progress book and badges awarded under *British Gymnastics* for both gymnastics and trampolining. The classes are very relaxed and informal with a short 'circle time' at the beginning and the end, which allows for lots of free play with parental assistance on the high beams and trampolines. My two boys have both enjoyed Gympups from 18 months and my eldest is still loving it at three and a half. The classes after this age are parent-free and carers can watch from the balcony above. There is a different theme each week, e.g. jumping, climbing, and rolling.'
Marguerite, mum of David and Dylan

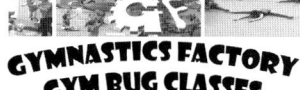

GYMNASTICS FACTORY GYM BUG CLASSES

Themed structured preschool gymnastics classes

from 4 months - 4 years
Fun Action packed sessions

The best way to encourage physical development

FOR DETAILS VISIT OUR WEBSITE
www.gymnasticsfactory.co.uk
01483 455 060

'The classes start with a singing warm-up then the children are 'let loose'. Each week there is a theme and the apparatus is set up in different ways. Emily enjoys using all of the equipment, which includes beams, bars, ladders, tunnels, balls, small trampolines, stepping stones, wobble boards, and she particularly enjoys her turn on the big trampoline. The staff are very friendly and help the children work towards Gympups and trampolining badges, for which they collect stickers. It is a really fun class and wonderful exercise.'
Angela, mum of Sophie and Emily

Tumble Tots
(01483) 420741
www.tumbletots.com
Godalming Masonic Hall – Mon and Tues
Guildford Girl Guide HQ, Nightingale Road – Wed
Scouts Hall, Ontario Way, Liphook – Thurs
The Arbuthnot Hall, Shamley Green – Fri
[Term-time: Class times vary according

Things to Do

to age (from six months to seven years). Trial class available, then payment per half term in advance. Also available for parties – see p174]

'I first took Dominic to Tumble Tots when he was eight months old, he is four and a half now and he still loves it. He can walk backwards across beams, do 'roly-polies', and climb everything with confidence. Laura started going when she could walk and she loves 'Tots, Tots' too.

Equipment is set out like an obstacle course and includes tunnels, beams, and climbing frames, which get bigger as the children get older. The session includes catchy songs at beginning and end; for younger ones classes are informal and include free play with sticks, bean bags, etc. It becomes more structured as child gets older. Very friendly helpers.'
Helen, mum of Dominic and Laura

'*Tumble Tots* comes to Guildford on Wednesdays with 45-minute sessions for one to five-year-olds throughout the day. The helpers are all really friendly, the atmosphere is always light hearted. James loves going and has gained so much confidence from using the equipment.'
Sally, mum of James

Woking Gymnastics Club
Kingfield Road
Woking
GU22 9AA
(01483) 771426
info@woking-gymnastics.co.uk
www.woking-gymnastics.co.uk
[See also 'Holiday Activities']

'Sessions start with a short warm-up, then the kids are let loose on modified but proper gym equipment. The beam has lots of soft blocks surrounding it to making walking practice safer. There is a baby swing from the men's high rings, and a slide is set up to land in a foam pit. There are things to walk on, under, and crawl through; a proper trampoline, and qualified gym teachers to help the kids and parents along the way.

There is another short cool down session with songs at the end. It is vast (to accommodate full size floor area). There are classes for a variety of ages on different days of the week, so it's good for mums who work part-time.'
Maggie, mum of Alice and Katy

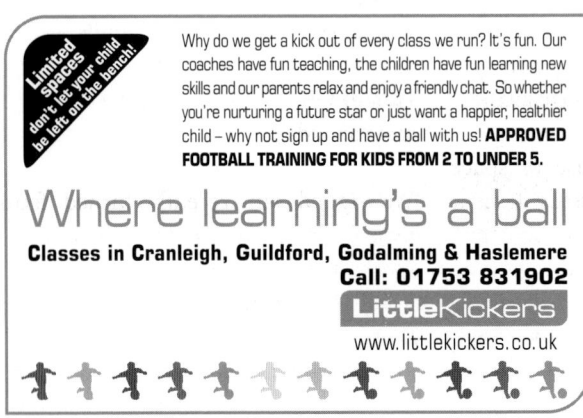

'*Woking Gymnastics Club* is bursting with energy, talent and runs some of the best gym classes in the area. It offers classes for boys and girls, from crawlers upwards. The club also develops top national gymnasts. Courses run every week day, every 45 minutes, from 9.30 am to 3.30 pm for preschoolers and from 3.45 pm for older children. The classes are really good fun, creative and cover the national curriculum using colours, numbers and shapes. There are also both non-structured and structured classes to introduce discipline. Gymnastics is great for my kids because it helps hand to eye co-ordination, balance, spatial awareness and is a fundamental grounding for all sports.'
Jo, mum of Lucy and Milly

Trampolining

Tots Trampolining (up to five years)
Sports Centre
University of Surrey
GU2 7XH
(01483) 689201
www.unisport.co.uk
Term-time: Friday 11.00 am – 12.00 pm
[Also see website for details of many other children's activities for school-age kids]

'Children just love the sense of space and freedom in this enormous hall; it is heaven, let them run! They can climb on the beams, play football, use the toys etc., and there are two big trampolines! There are lots of student helpers from the university trampolining club who encourage kids to use correct techniques, but it's very informal so no pressure. Four children are supervised on each trampoline at a time, so there's not usually much waiting for turns. The session ends with the *Hokey Cokey*. Try to get there a bit early as the car park can get busy and has very narrow spaces; you also need to get a flyer from the sports centre reception to put on your windscreen. There's no need to book in advance, just turn up.'
Helen, mum of Dominic and Laura

'It is well run, has two trampolines, climbing bars, and other gym equipment for the little ones to play with, such as balls and hoops. At the end of each session the leader gathers everyone together to sing the '*Hokey Cokey*' to get rid of the last drop of toddler energy. Very reasonably priced too.'
Jacqui, mum of Harry and Megan

Trampolining
Guildford Spectrum Leisure Complex
Parkway
GU1 1UP
(01483) 443322
www.guildfordspectrum.co.uk
Term-time: Wednesday 4.15 – 5.15 pm; Saturday 9.30 – 10.30 am (for four to six-year-olds)

'We signed our recently turned four-year-old son up for this class as he enjoys bouncing on his grandparents' trampoline. The staff are very attentive, patient and skilled, but the discipline of learning new movements is a little demanding for one so young. I feel the

Things to Do

class is a little too structured for his age; it aims to teach techniques, and time on the trampoline is limited.'
David, dad of Harry

Football

Chelsea Indoor Football Coaching
*Guildford Spectrum Leisure Complex
Parkway
GU1 1UP
(01483) 443322
www.guildfordspectrum.co.uk*
Term-time: Monday 4.00 pm (for four to five-year-olds)

'This [Mini Kicking] class is run by football development officers employed by *Chelsea Football Club*. The class is fun but still incorporates skills/techniques of the game. The first half-hour usually comprises chase and tag games with a ball, followed by mini-matches divided into age groups.

Most of the kids seem to enjoy it and the teachers are sympathetic, fairly gentle and engender a fun environment. They know when to add a bit of discipline and also are aware of their responsibilities when dealing with young children. You can also view from the 'gallery' above so you see everything but don't get in the way! Recommended – particularly in the winter!'
David, dad of Harry

Little Kickers
*(01753) 831902
www.littlekickers.co.uk*
Wilfrid Noyce Centre – Friday 3.30 pm and 4.30 pm; Guildford Grove School – Sat 9.30 am and 11.00 am; Merrow Village Hall – Sun 10.30 am, 11.00 am and 12.00 pm
[Class times are age-dependent. Plus other venues all over Surrey – see website or phone for details; Runs 50 weeks a year]

'*Little Kickers* is a fun, confidence-building introduction to football for the under-fives. There is a lot of emphasis on general exercise and games as well as scoring 'super big goals.' Parents take a book or paper and let the coaches get the children exercised and appetites built up for lunch.'
Alex, dad of Dominic and Laura

Socatots
*2 Pewtrees Cottages
Lower Eashing
Godalming
GU7 2QD
(01483) 416002
guildford@socatots.com
www.socatots.com/guildford*

[Classes run in Surrey every day at 9.30 am and 10.15 am, and all day on Saturday. See website for venues and sessions. Class times are age-dependent]

Tennis

Mini Tennis Academy
Guildford Spectrum Leisure Complex
Parkway
GU1 1UP
(01483) 443322
www.guildfordspectrum.co.uk
[Term-time: run in association with *TENNIStogether* for children aged three to ten. Ring the *Spectrum* for details]

Ice Skating

Parent & Toddler Skate
Also held at Guildford Spectrum (see above)
Term-time: Monday – Friday
12.00 – 4.00 pm
[Special price rates for adults with children under five years]

Ice Pups
Also held at Guildford Spectrum (see above)
Monday and Wednesday 4.15 – 4.45 pm
Thursday 2.10 – 2.40 pm
[Term-time courses for children aged three to five years teaching basic skating moves and confidence through fun and play]

Swimming

Swimming is a fun activity for carer and child alike, and is invaluable for building confidence in the water. This section is spilt between 'swimming lessons' and 'informal swimming'. The 'swimming lessons' usually require pre-booking and may have a waiting list, so please contact the swimming pool/class in advance. Most operate during term-time only and usually require payment in advance, either termly or half-termly. If you choose to attend one of the 'informal swimming' entries, you can turn up as and when you desire.

Swimming Lessons

Aquaschool
Guildford lessons based at:
Lockwood Centre
Slyfield Industrial Estate
GU1 1RR
(01483) 306964
www.aquaschool.co.uk
[Lessons from three months]

'Jessica has really grown to love being underwater as a result of these swimming lessons. The lessons are held at the Lockwood pool on the Slyfield estate, and parking is always difficult. Other downsides are the small changing rooms which can get very cramped. However, the pool is really warm, and the tutors and the babies' fun and development make the effort and cost worthwhile.

Guildford NCT has much to offer

- ❖ Antenatal and refresher classes
- ❖ Early days postnatal courses
- ❖ New to...social and informative get-togethers
- ❖ Bumps and babes
- ❖ Coffees, teas and socials
- ❖ Nearly new sales
- ❖ Swimming at the Spectrum
- ❖ Breastfeeding support
- ❖ Breast pump hire
- ❖ NCT bras
- ❖ Valley cushion hire
- ❖ Branch library
- ❖ Local and national experience registers
- ❖ Quarterly newsletter

To find out more call: (0870) 4609631
email: *info@nctguildford.org.uk* or
see: *www.nctguildford.org.uk*

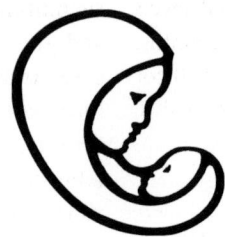

Each term lasts nine sessions, and follows the school term-timetable. Early booking advised, particularly for levels one and two.'
Heather, mum of Jessica

Baby Swimming
Guildford lessons based at:
Lockwood Centre
Slyfield Industrial Estate
GU1 1RR
(01865) 794222
info@babyswimming.co.uk
www.babyswimming.co.uk
[Babies can join these classes up until the age of 14 months. Once started, they can continue until they are three and a half]

'Ella started when she was ten months old but they take babies a lot younger. The advantages of these classes are they are small in numbers and the pool use is restricted for the classes and therefore quieter than public pools. The temperature is in the thirties, which is lovely in winter but rather hot in summer. The teachers are excellent and Ella loves her weekly session.'
Lynn, mum of Ella

'My 16 month old has completed levels one to four over the last 12 months. The courses cost just under £100.00 for a nine week course, which is expensive, particularly if you miss sessions, as we have, due to coughs, colds etc. However, we have really enjoyed the lessons, where babies are introduced to being splashed, dunked, swimming underwater, holding onto the side of the pool and jumping in off the side. Not only has my son enjoyed the lessons, I have also learned a lot about how to help him develop his swimming skills.

On the downside, the classes can feel quite rushed as there are usually other groups using the pool before and after your class. Also, the changing rooms aren't great and there is a shortage of parking for the weekday classes. However, the pool is heated to a balmy 32 degrees, and I have some great underwater photos of my son, which make these minor hassles worthwhile.'
Louise, mum of James

'Swimming from three months to three or four years. Babies are introduced to swimming underwater where it's apparently easier to swim and, don't worry, at a very early age babies have a flap that closes over their windpipe. It's best to introduce your baby at a very early age, as the later you leave it the more independent they become, and they protest at being laid on their back in the water. Classes are for up to nine children, each supported by a parent in the pool.

I took my daughter through the swimming lessons right up to four years and she now has a love of water and great confidence. She's having to learn the swimming strokes elsewhere, but has the all important confidence. Not cheap (£98.00 for 9 lessons) but you are giving your child a wonderful life-skill. One other small benefit for *Baby Swimming* is that if your child is ill and has to miss a

Things to Do

class you can do two catch up classes per term on another day.'
Sonya, mum of Eleanor and Charles

Aqua Tots
(0208) 6886488
info@aquatots.com
www.aquatots.com
[For babies from ten weeks to six years. Classes available in Guildford, Ottershaw, Leatherhead, Farnborough and other locations]

Aqua Pups
Guildford Spectrum Leisure Complex
Parkway
GU1 1UP
(01483) 443322
www.guildfordspectrum.co.uk

Term-time course: Friday 9.30 – 10.00 am [Half-hour structured learn-to-swim programme. For children aged five months to four years. Pay-per-session]

'Freya and I went swimming for the first time today and it was fabulous. A half-hour session cost £4.60 and we had two members of staff facilitating with noodles, floats, toys and songs. A very enjoyable outing.'
Colleen, mum of Freya

Duckling Club
Also held at Guildford Spectrum (see above)
(01483) 562900 (Emma Bunce)
Term-time: Thursday and Friday 12.00 – 1.30 pm. [Swimming sessions for parents and under-fours.]

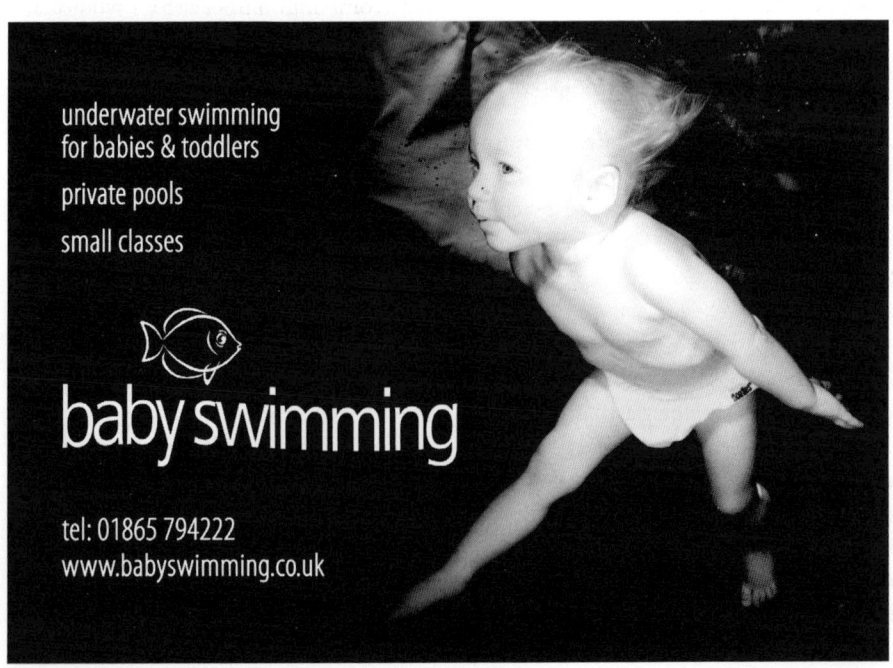

underwater swimming for babies & toddlers
private pools
small classes

baby swimming

tel: 01865 794222
www.babyswimming.co.uk

'Part of the teaching pool is cordoned off and filled with different sized toys including balls, ducks, boats, etc. There is a dedicated lifeguard to the *'Ducklings'* and a friendly instructor, so one parent can take two children. The instructor will help you and your baby in and out of the pool, and gives you ideas to help your child swim. There are changing mats at the side of the pool for babies, so you can get them changed just before you get in and get out. Grandparents are welcome. You can do a trial session, then pay half-termly in advance. Good value for money.'
Mary, mum of Jack, Charlie, Chloe and Georgia

Guildford NCT Swim Sessions
Also held at Guildford Spectrum (see above)
(01483) 574650 (Alison Curtis)
Term-time: Tuesday 1.30 – 3.30 pm
[For parents and under-fours. Held in training pool. £13.00 per half term or £25.00 per term; £3.00 trial session deducted from term cost. See also entry under All About the NCT p7]

'A great way of introducing water to your baby. Floats are available. Plenty of toys in the pool for baby to play with and an instructor/supervisor is on hand at all times as well as a lifeguard. Baby can be dressed/changed easily as there are plenty of changing mats beside the pool. First visit is £3.00, then if you join half-term prices start at £13.00. Changing rooms are good with baby-changing pods and baby seats for while you change.'
Anna, mum of Logan

Woking NCT Swim Sessions
Woking Pool in the Park
Kingfield Road
Woking
GU22 9BA
(01483) 771122
poolinthepark@woking.gov.uk
www.woking.gov.uk
(01483) 824067 (Katherine Cunningham);
(01932) 340715 (Caroline Cackett)
Term-time: Monday 3.00 pm;
Wednesday 10.30 am, 1.30 pm and 2.00 pm [£3.50 per session]

'We've been taking our son to the *Pool in The Park* in Woking since he was a baby and now at five, he still loves it there. There are three pools – a shallow, warm and relatively quiet teaching pool, a 25-metre competition pool and a fun Leisure Lagoon, complete with waves, slides and rapids. The changing rooms are spacious and clean, with plenty of family changing rooms and baby-change tables. There's a good café upstairs that sells basic food, snacks and drinks, and we've always been able to get a table there after our swim.'
Julie, mum of Ben and Katie

Jan Harley Swim School
Esporta Health and Fitness Club
Queen Elizabeth Park
Railton Road
(01483) 540250
janharley@msn.com
www.esporta.com

'Although only for members' children, these classes are definitely worth joining the gym for. Jan as a teacher was recommended to me, and my daughter Freyja (aged four) loves the classes. When she started she was afraid of the water and being on her own with the instructor. After the second session she was much more confident and is now swimming and enjoying it.

The classes are small, only four per class at the most. There are several classes and levels, including private lessons. The emphasis is on having fun as well as learning to swim. The parents do not participate but can either watch from the pool side or have a swim themselves. The pool is relatively small, clean, warm and luxurious.

Definitely worth a look for members and those thinking of joining (you just need off-peak membership).'
Thora, mum of Frejya

Esporta Club – Childcare Facilities

'While *Esporta* itself is not well equipped for babies and small toddlers, it has negotiated a deal with the neighbouring *Kids Inc* nursery for two hour sessions: 9.30 – 11.30 am and 1.30 – 1.30 pm for £9.00 per session. *Kids Inc* offers free taster sessions to make sure your child settles and you're happy with the care provided.

Esporta/Kids Inc sessions do not include provision of meals, but the staff are happy to give bottles if you provide them. Sessions need to be booked in advance to ensure availability.'
Heather, mum of Jessica

Pool in the Park
Woking Park
Kingfield Road
Woking
GU22 9BA
(01483) 771122
poolinthepark@woking.gov.uk
www.woking.gov.uk
[Range of classes according to age. Approximately £4.50 for half-hour session for *Woking Borough* residents and £5.20 for non-residents. Paid termly.]

'I have been very impressed by the standard of the tuition of the swimming teachers. The classes start with nursery rhymes to encourage water confidence along with swimming position at an early age. My eldest son has progressed from 'Ducks' through to Beginners level 1, and he is now beginning to swim a few strokes without arm bands. Initially the waiting list for lessons is extremely long, however. I put both my sons' names down on the list practically from birth. Once you are in the system you always get a place at the next level. If you can get your under two-year-old's name down, it is well worth it.'
Chloe, mum of Conor and Anton

The Herons Swimming and Fitness Centre
Kings Road
Haslemere
GU27 2QA
(01428) 658484
enquiries@theheronsswimandfitnesscentre.co.uk
www.dcleisurecentres.co.uk

Things to Do

'*The Herons* has a good range of facilities, which include two pools, soft play, café, gym and crèche. George has been thoroughly enjoying swimming lessons here since he was three years old. The junior pool is a nice temperature and there are plenty of family cubicles in the changing rooms. Lessons are available for mother and baby right through to older children.'
Nicki, mum of George and Olivia

The Swimming Academy
Zelda Glasspell
25 Highfield Path
Cove
GU14 0HN
(01252) 512981
www.theswimmingacademy.com
zelda@theswimmingacademy.com
Classes held in Guildford (Lockwood centre and Boxgrove Primary School), Godalming, Camberley and Farnham. Classes from 5 months to adult.

Informal Swimming

Bracknell Leisure Centre Swimming Pool
Bagshot Road
Bracknell
RG12 9SE
(01344) 454203
www.bracknell-forest.gov.uk/leisure

'Highly rated by Ella's dad as clean, warm pool and decent changing room facilities.'
Leena, mum of Ella

Coral Reef - Bracknell's Water World
Nine Mile Ride
Bracknell
RG12 7JQ
(01344) 862525
www.bracknell-forest.gov.uk/coralreef

'*Coral Reef* is a wonderful 'waterworld' for kids and adults alike. The first thing you notice is the enormous ship in the water, which my little boy thought was great. There is a large freeform swimming pool which has a wave machine at regular intervals, a 'lazy river', a few waterfalls, and on the other side of one of them you can swim outside. There are also several water chutes, one of which is family-friendly – you can go down with a toddler on your lap. I haven't visited 'sauna world' – my kids are too young but it all looks lovely – calm and relaxed. In addition to the saunas, there are sunbeds, a Japanese steam room, a large spa pool, and a sunken foot spa. You can even use the gym or visit the sauna world café. You can get adequate refreshments at *Coconut Grove*.'
Emma, mum of Charlotte and Louis

Guildford Lido
Stoke Rd
Guildford
GU1 1HB
(01483) 444888
www.guildford.gov.uk/GuildfordWeb/Leisure/SportsFacilities/GuildfordLido
[Open May to September 10.30 am – 6.30 pm for public swimming; adult-only

lane-swim Tuesday and Thursday 7.00 – 8.40 pm; during July pool opening times may vary due to school swimming galas – check website or call for details; £4.50 for adults (all day); £3.50 after 4.30 pm]

'The *Lido* is a great place to spend a warm summer's day. There are large grassy lawns, with some trees on the hill that give off enough shade for the babies. There is a long shallow paddling pool and a 50m heated (though still quite chilly!) outdoor pool which is lovely for a swim – we would go in a group and take turns watching the babies while we swam laps. Picnics are welcome, but there is a snack bar that serves burgers, chips, ice cream, etc. There are outdoor toilets, showers, and stalls for adult changing, but I don't remember any specific baby-changing – we would just change them on the lawn. There is also crazy golf but I've never tried that.'
Kelley, mum of Audrey

Guildford Spectrum Leisure Complex
Parkway
GU1 1UP
(01483) 443322
www.guildfordspectrum.co.uk

Spectrum Leisure Pool
[at non-toddler splash times]

'We often take our children swimming late on a Friday afternoon or on a Saturday morning. While it can be busy, they don't seem to mind. There is plenty there to enjoy, including the wave machine, pirate ship, fountains and slides. Some of the smaller slides they can do by themselves, but it is a lot of fun taking them down on our laps on the larger flumes. There are large family changing rooms in addition to the usual individual cubicles. The *Spectrum* does have a rule that children under four must be accompanied by an adult on a one-to-one ratio. The café is good for post-swim drinks and snacks.'
Alison, mum of Laura and Daniel

'At the weekend, *Spectrum*'s Teaching Pool opens 30 minutes before the Leisure Pool and is great for those with very small children and babies. (It's also slightly cheaper so better value for short visits). Unfortunately once your little one discovers the delights of the Leisure Pool there is usually no turning back. Early mornings are less crowded and Sunday mornings are designated 'family time'. Afternoons can involve queuing (when the pool reaches capacity), and in the winter the changing area floor can get a little mucky over the course of the day.

The water temperature and changing rooms can be a little cold, but my daughter never minds once she's in the water and if you keep a towel by the side of the pool and play a 'how fast can you dress' game it's usually not a problem. There are family changing rooms and hairdryers available. After swimming my daughter loves to go to the coffee shop – but be prepared for a queue. To pass the time I usually bring a drink or snack for my daughter to start while we queue.'
Sandra, mum of Eloise

Spectrum Toddler Splash
Held at Guildford Spectrum (see above)
[Exclusively for adults with under-fives]
Term-time: Tuesday and Thursday 10.30 am – 12.00 pm (ring to check – session sometimes does not run in the weeks either side of school holidays.)

'*Toddler Splash* is great! If you get there on time, you'll be the first in the changing rooms so it's always easy to find a cubicle and the floor is nice and dry (very important with a toddler that likes to chuck the contents of your bag on the floor!) There are also some large family changing rooms to make life easier, and for smaller babies, baby seats fastened to the walls are provided so that you can keep them safe while you change.

During the session the leisure pool is reserved just for babies and toddlers, so it's a fab way to introduce them to the water. My toddler loves discovering all the different pools and animals in the water. The staff switch on different fountains and bubble sections at different times, so there is always something new to look at. The best bit for overgrown children like me is that they have one of the big slides open, and you can take your toddler down on your lap.

Towards the end of the session they switch the wave machine on. Afterwards you can go upstairs for the all important coffee and cake!'
Jo, mum of Stanley

'We all love T*oddler Splash*, the fountains, slides and pirate ship. It's special because it is the only time one adult is allowed to take two under-fours swimming (all other times under-fours need to be accompanied on a one adult to one child basis). Take a £1.00 coin for the lockers. For real thrill-seekers you can get a reduced rate T*oddler Splash* and soft play combo ticket.'
Helen, mum of Dominic and Laura

Horsham Pavilions in the Park
Hurst Road
Horsham
RH12 2DF
(01403) 219200
www.thepavilionsinthepark.co.uk

'Swimming pools are interlinked and include a heated outdoor pool. Although a bit of a trek, it's worth it if you then use the children's play park as well, which is large and full of activities, lovely on a summer's day.'
Leena, mum of Ella

Woking Parent and Toddler Splash
Woking Pool in the Park
Kingfield Road
Woking
GU22 9BA
(01483) 771122
poolinthepark@woking.gov.uk
www.woking.gov.uk
Term-time: Monday, Wednesday and Friday 11.00 – 11.45 am or 11.45 am –12.30 pm; Sunday: 9.15 – 10.00 am (time may vary during state school holidays)
[Capacity: Sessions are limited to a maximum of 36 swimmers in the pool]

Things to Do

Soft Play

Soft play areas seem to be an almost compulsory part of childhood these days. They are fantastic big padded areas where children from crawling age can practise cruising, climbing, building and turning around, and older ones can take off at top speed and work up a good sweat even in the depths of winter. Soft play is a much more flexible option than clubs or classes, and is useful in cold/wet weather or as a venue to meet friends when the front room gets too small for all eight toddlers from your antenatal class. Many have a separate area for the under-fours with larger apparatus for older children. Often there are refreshments available, which in many cases are getting better and better in quality and 'child-friendly' food. The disadvantages are that most get incredibly busy during the school holidays, or after school hours during term-time; otherwise they can be a heaven-sent place to take the children to burn off some energy indoors. Don't forget to always take socks for both you and the kids even in the summer. It is worth mentioning that of course your children are your responsibility at all times.

Crazy Tots
Leatherhead Leisure Centre car park
Guildford Road
Fetcham
Leatherhead
KT22 9BL
(01372) 377718
www.leatherheadleisurecentre.co.uk
Monday – Friday 9.30 am – 4.30 pm (10.00 am – 4.30 pm during school holidays)
Saturday and Sunday 9.30 am – 12.30 pm

'*Crazy Tots* is a soft play area inside Leatherhead Leisure Centre, about a half-hour drive from Guildford. There is a small soft play area with wobbly bridge and a slide into the ball pit which even the younger toddlers can manage and then a really big soft area with all sorts of shapes for climbing/sliding on, and a big bouncy castle. Can get busy during the school holidays and at weekends. I found this a great place to take two toddlers as it is very open and both can be seen at all times! There is also an area with changing mats in the pram park, and toilets are close by. Lots of free parking available at the leisure centre but allow about five minutes to get from the car to the *Crazy Tots* play area as it's a bit of a walk.'
Marguerite, mum of David and Dylan

'The soft play area ('*Crazy Tots*'), located in a gymnasium, is huge, with lots of clambering, climbing and jumping equipment, including a ball pit and full-size bouncy castle! Great for babies and up to five years. There is a bench all along one side where mums can watch and chat, a small area for non-walkers;

and the leisure centre café serves decent, reasonably priced food. Less climbing frame-like than *Specky's Pirate Ship* or *Little Angels*. It has saved my sanity many a time, but is better avoided in school holidays. Also – always call before you go, to check it's open, as sometimes the area is closed for special sporting events.'
Paige, mum of Miranda and Leo

Farncombe Fun Zone
(formerly the **Cool Club**)
The Warehouse
Owen Road
Farncombe
Godalming
GU7 3AY
(01483) 861666
Monday to Saturday 10.00 am – 5.30 pm; Sunday 11.00 am – 5.00 pm
[Six months to ten years. See also under Services – 'Parties' p167]

'I have just discovered this place with a group of NCT mums. We have toddlers and crawlers and the place is fantastic. It is soft play with a ball pool, slides, tunnels and climbing equipment. You can always see the toddlers as the place is quite small. There is also a separate area for babies, which is easy to see while you watch the toddlers at the same time. Very friendly and courteous staff. Good menu for food with adult and child portions. Child-friendly toilets and changing area. All very clean and tidy. A great place to spend a couple of hours.'
Jane, mum of Jessica

'This is a fantastic soft play for younger children. It is our favourite one and we go at least once a week. What I like about this soft play is that it is relatively small and cosy without being claustrophobic. There is a separate baby area and the seating area is comfortable and clean. There is an extensive menu and healthy snacks on offer. The staff are friendly and this is a family run business. Freyja had her second birthday party here and we have been to many there since. Definitely worth it for those looking to 'outsource' their child's birthday party. Prices are reasonable.'
Thora, mum of Freyja

'Great soft play for preschoolers – even my five-year-old still finds it fun. Smaller and less busy than other soft play areas. Food isn't great but it is cheap. Car park is quite small so you may have to find a parking spot on the road. The staff are very friendly and friends say that they do good parties there.'
Rachel, mum of Amy, Thomas and Ella

Fizzy Kids
10 Camp Road
Farnborough
GU14 6EW
(01252) 669977
www.fizzykids.co.uk

'*Fizzy Kids* is good fun. There is a really big play frame for older children, and a surprisingly large, fun-packed and enclosed play area for younger ones. However, you can't easily see one area from another, which is a downside for me, as I like to able to see both my children, or at least have easy access to them.

The café is pretty good, reasonably priced and has a lovely lunch box choice for children, although, again you can't easily see most of the larger play frame from the café. And the toilet facilities are generally clean and well maintained. A fun trip out, but rather a lot of trekking around to check up on the kids.'
Emma, mum of Charlotte and Louis

'A medium-sized soft play that is clean and great for kids from crawlers upwards. There is comfortable seating within an under-fours area. Air conditioning is great in summer. Healthy food is available for parents and children. We had our son's party here and it was well organized and stress free. There are two car parks in walking distance and on-street parking outside.'
Rachel, mum of Amy, Thomas and Ella

Gym Jams
Normandy Village Hall
Manor Fruit Farm
Glaziers Lane
Normandy
GU3 2DE
(01932) 340379 (Barry or Millie)
info@gym-jams.co.uk
www.gym-jams.co.uk
Wednesday 9.30 – 11.00 am; 11.15 am – 12.45 pm; 1.00 – 2.30 pm; Friday 9.30 – 11.30 am [Sessions run all year round. See 'Holiday Activities' p65]

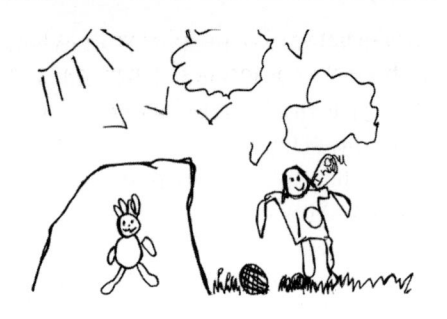

'We love these soft play sessions. There are loads of play areas for pre-walkers as well as for little tots. As *Gym Jams* is only for children from 0 to four, I find it a little bit more suitable for my toddler than other soft play places, as it has more activities for his age group. There is a bouncy castle, a trampoline, a ball pool, a slide and loads of tunnels to go through and discover. Everything is always very clean, including the toilets and changing facilities. You get a drink and biscuit for your child included in the entrance price. There are several sessions on a Wednesday and one on Friday morning.'
Nadine, mum of Noah and Luca

'A really great soft play set-up in a large, modern, clean and airy village hall. There is a big bouncy castle in one corner and all the usual ball pits and soft play equipment in the rest of the hall. There are baby gyms and mats for the very young. You can get a drink part way through the session, which runs for an hour and a half. The only down side is that the sessions are set times, so you need to find one that suits you and

they're not pre-bookable, so you just have to hope it's not too busy when you turn up. Apparently you can get turned away if it's full - it's first come, first served – so make sure you arrive promptly!'
Charlotte, mum of Karina

'Great as a regular meeting place. You can feed the babies/children, meet up with other mums and let the little ones enjoy a great play. Lots of toys for all ages. Also great as a 'filler' when the weather isn't great.'
Avril, mum of Scarlett

Jakes
2B London Road
Bagshot
GU19 5HN
(01276) 453555
www.jakesplayworld.co.uk
jakesplayworld@yahoo.co.uk

'Soft play frame with ball canons, big slide, mini indoor football/basketball pitch. In dry weather there is a small outdoor area with bouncy castle, water-play tables, wendy house, ride-on toys, tables for mums... There is a separate under-fours

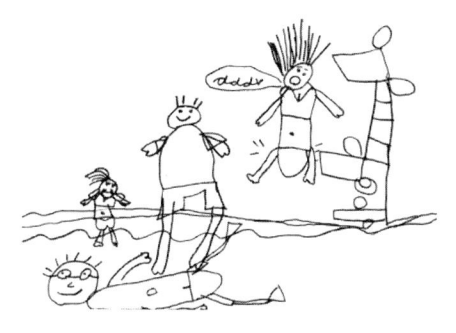

area. Check website for special events e.g. story times, children's discos, 'Messy Mondays' etc. Café available. There is a small car park, however if this is full you can also use *Pantiles* night club car park near by.'
Jo, mum of Marcus, Alex and Elizabeth

Rainbow Tots
Knaphill Scout Hall
Waterers Rise
Knaphill
Woking
GU21 2HU
(07803) 600720 (Angela Sanderson)
(07885) 702414 (Hazel Stevens)
info@rainbowtots.com
www.rainbowtots.com
Term-time: Tuesday and Wednesday 10.00 am – 2.30 pm;
Friday 10.00 am – 2.30 pm
[Check website for school holiday times, See 'Holiday Activities' p66]

'A perfect way to spend a weekday with others. Good facilities and plenty of toys for all ages. Younger toddlers will be excited at trying out things they don't have at home. A great place to drop in when you want a local and friendly soft play! Very friendly and helpful when looking for directions.'
Avril, mum of Scarlett

'An excellent soft play centre for mums to meet other mums and for babies to let off some steam. A cordoned off area for younger babies/non-crawlers, and an excellent array of ride-ons for those

Things to Do

wanting a bit more excitement. There are some small indoor playground/park activities as well, e.g. see-saw, and there is a bouncy castle for older children. Great tea/coffee facilities available.'
Anna, mum of Logan

Roker's Little Angels
Fairlands Farm
Aldershot Road
Guildford
GU3 3PB
(01483) 236667
Open daily 9.30 am – 6.30 pm [Six months to 11 years.]

'*Little Angels* is big, and open every day, so pre-booking is not required. The main play area is dominated by a large multi-lane slide and climbing area for the older children. There is also a separate play area for the under-fours, with a ball pool and a smaller climbing area, which is nice if you have little ones. There are plenty of tables and highchairs and a small café that does basic food and drinks for adults and children. There is a changing room.'
Kelley, mum of Audrey

'A large indoor soft play with two separate areas. One is for under-fours only, and the much larger main area is for children old enough to want to venture inside it (about 20 months in our case), although the younger ones will probably need accompanying. Tons of different things to do with all the usual soft play equipment: climbing, tunnels, slides (the main central slide is for the over-fours only), ball pools, rope swings plus a 'scary' blackout area. A number of other 'pay-as-you-go' ride-ons are dotted around the place too. There are plenty of highchairs and the usual selection of food on offer in the café.'
Lisa, mum of Thomas

'Great soft play area for toddlers, including a ball pit, stairs and lots of shapes to climb on/over/move around. The baby area is away from the older children's play area, so it feels safe. Drinks and snacks are available, and there are tables and chairs for parents to supervise from.'
Heather, mum of Jessica

Runabout Indoor Soft Play Centre
Armstrong Way
The Fairway
Ively Road
Farnborough
GU14 0LP
(01252) 370721
www.run-about.co.uk

'Although this soft play is a little further away than some (about 30 minutes drive from Guildford) it is well worth the effort. I started coming here when my small toddlers outgrew the baby areas of other more local soft play places but were not yet big enough to go up to the three or four storey zones! This one really bridged the gap and is ideal for the 18 months to four years age group. There is a small area for infants, a ball pit for the under-fives, a spacious area with ride-ons and play houses, as well as the main soft play zone. My two-year-old son was safe to go round

on his own as there are no large drops, just one medium slide to watch for but he soon mastered it! The area is surrounded by plenty of comfy sofas and tables and chairs so you can choose a good vantage point to watch your children. There is a good variety of hot and cold food served including organic options. The only downside is that it is quite hidden away so make sure you know exactly where you are going – take a map for the first few visits!'
Alison, mum of Laura and Daniel

Rushmoor Gym
The Gymnastics Centre
Pool Road
Aldershot
GU11 3SN
(01252) 320888 (Colin and Bernie Wright)
info@rushgym.co.uk
www.rushgym.co.uk
Term-time: Playgym sessions 9.30 – 10.30 am and 1.30 – 2.30 pm; £1.00 per person Also holiday Playgym – see website.
[See also 'Gymnastics' p24 and 'Holiday Activities' p66]

'If you don't mind the journey, this gym is fantastic. There are two daily pay-as-you-go sessions for five years and under, these sessions are a bargain price and worth the drive over from Guildford. The gymnasium is full of equipment and space for running around. There is a bouncy castle and the trampolines are at floor level making it slightly less stressful for parents.'
Thora, mum of Freyja

'This a fantastic place to take your child to run off some energy. You have access to all the professional gym equipment – beams, trampolines and even ride-on cars and a bouncy castle. It is suitable for 0 to fives and offers everyone the opportunity to run wild for an hour! Well worth the trip – easy parking outside the gym. No café but does have a drinks machine.'
Rebecca, mum of Isabelle, Aimee and Robyn

Specky's Pirate Ship
Guildford Spectrum Leisure Complex
Parkway
GU1 1UP
(01483) 443322
www.guildfordspectrum.co.uk
Monday – Wednesday 9.30 am – 5.00 pm; Thursday and Friday 9.30 am – 3.30 pm (unless there are no parties, in which case it's open later); Saturday and Sunday 9.00 am – 12.00 pm. Up to ten years

'This soft play area is spread over three floors and is an excellent way of exercising little legs. There is a variety of areas for the inquisitive mind and Ella loves sitting in the ball areas and going down the slides. There are large foam steps between levels that are too big for small children to climb so it keeps you fit carrying them up and down! Toilets and coffee facilities are not within this area but there are lockers to keep valuables.'
Lynn, mum of Ella

'Highly rated by Ella's dad as a place to take a two-year-old when instructed to

Things to Do

let mum have 'mum time'. Saturday and Sunday mornings are usually nice and quiet.'
Leena, mum of Ella

Toad Hall
Goldsworth Lodge
Goldsworth Park
Woking
GU21 3RT
(01483) 799700
elaine.sayers@toadhall-nursery.co.uk
www.toadhall-nursery.co.uk
10.00 am – 6.00 pm seven days a week, closing occasionally for private parties

'This was one of the first ever play zones opened. It is a huge play frame with several storeys. Several spiral slides, including a spooky dark one. There is a good baby section, which is <u>free</u> to non-walkers. There is a coffee shop which serves a range of snacks and drinks. There is a disabled toilet with nappy changing facilities.'
Chloe, mum of Conor and Anton

Wizzy World
The Big Purple Building
6 Invincible Road
Farnborough
GU14 7QU
(0845) 226 2329
www.wizzy-world.com
9.30 am – 6.00 pm seven days a week

'*Wizzy World* is my favourite soft play. The play area itself is within a really large frame, with all sorts of climbing, dodging, balancing, squeezing and sliding activities. It's also big enough for me to get in without feeling really claustrophobic. I like it because there are comfortable sofas everywhere, and because the big soft play area is designed so that you can almost always see your child. There is also a smaller play frame for younger children. This is enclosed, so they can't escape. You can also sit within this area on one of the many comfy sofas, and still see the larger play area pretty well.

The toilets are clean, with smaller toilets and sinks for 'littlies'. There is a separate disabled toilet with a baby-changer. The café provides reasonably priced food, which is pretty good, especially the kids' lunch boxes where they can have five items including very fresh sandwiches, sausages, crisps, cheese cubes, grapes, yoghurts, fruit juices etc. There are tables and chairs both downstairs and upstairs, and you can access the play frame from either level.'
Emma, mum of Charlotte and Louis

Pick'n'Mix Playstore
Woking Leisure Centre
Woking Park
Kingfield Road,
Woking
GU22 9BA
(01483) 771122
leisurecentre@woking.gov.uk
www.woking.gov.uk
Term-time: 11.00 am – 6.30 pm Monday – Friday; 9.30 am – 12.30 pm Saturday and Sunday – times subject to change during holidays. Call for details.

Mini sessions exclusively for 18 months to under-fives, parental supervision required, pre-booking recommended. All sessions take place in the *Pick'n'Mix Playstore* combined with a different activity every day. All include exclusive use of the *Playstore*, juice and biscuits:

- **Mini Bookworms**: Monday 10.00 – 10.45 am, *Playstore* combined with a story telling
- **Mini Mix**: Tuesday and Thursday 10.00 – 10.45 am, *Playstore* combined with colouring-in and nursery rhymes
- **Mini Telly Tots**: Wednesday 10.00 – 10.45 am, *Playstore* and a video
- **Mini Pop Tarts**: Friday 10.00 – 10.45 am, *Playstore* combined with a mini disco with lights and music

'We like this because it's really quiet (term-time and before schools finish). There is a separate under-fours area and the main area is quite easy to navigate. The main attraction is a curly slide that lands in a deep ball bit. The toilets and baby-changing are quite a walk away though. The park outside adjacent to the car park is good fun too if you fancy fresh air after.'
Sally, mum of James

'I visited *Pick'n'Mix Playstore* for the first time today during the under-fives Friday *Pop Tarts* session. I can't believe it has taken me so long to find this place. I strongly recommend a visit. We were the only ones there at first, I think it must be seriously under used in the mornings especially, so a great place to meet up with friends. It is huge, over several stories but quite easy to navigate for grown-ups. Both my four-year-old and two-year-old loved it. Especially the curly slide which has a tube next to it to post balls into. We will definitely go back.'
Helen, mum of Dominic and Laura

Soft Play
(Also held at Woking Leisure centre – see above, but different venue from Pick'n'Mix Playstore)
Monday 9.30 – 10.30 am, for age two to five years
Wednesday 9.30 – 10.30 am, for age 12 months to two years; 10.30 – 11.30 am, for age 12 months to two years

[Soft Play equipment with climbing apparatus and small bouncy castle. Parental supervision only. Includes singing and parachute if member of staff available.]

The Herons Swimming and Fitness Centre
Kings Road
Haslemere
GU27 2QT
(01428) 658484
enquiries@theheronsswimandfitnesscentre.co.uk
www.dcleisurecentres.co.uk

'Small soft play area with a coffee bar right next door. The sports centre also holds several other activities for under-fives during term-time, and then holiday activities for over fives.'
Nicki, mum of George and Olivia

Things to Do

Music Groups

Introducing children from a young age to the joys of music is important for their development. Within the Guildford area we are fortunate to have a number of music groups that are aimed at children under the age of five. So for all those budding musicians carry on reading and happy music-making!

Baby Bounce and Rhyme
Guildford Library
77 North Street
GU1 4AL
(08456) 009009
libraries@surreycc.gov.uk
www.surreycc.gov.uk
Tuesday 11.00 – 11.30 am
[Designed for babies up to one year, but ok for older siblings to attend.]

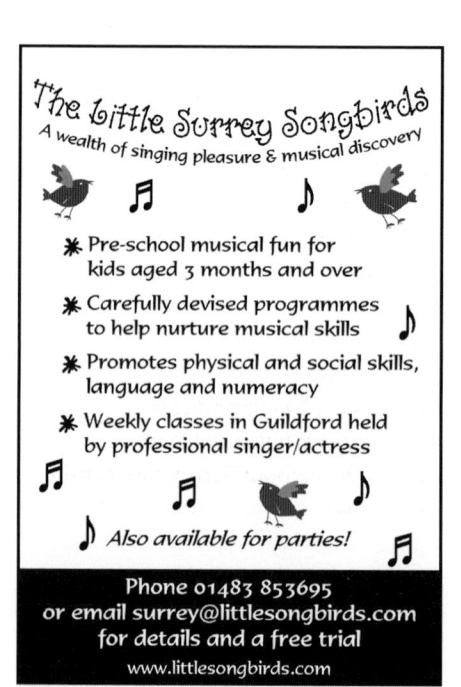

'This is a great freebie offered by the very helpful and enthusiastic library staff. The babies get their own book bag once they have been to six sessions. There are always lots of babies, at this excellent sing-a-long.'
Colleen, Mum of Freya

'This is a free activity, and although obviously very popular, it can be a bit daunting on your first visit as it is packed with children everywhere! It is very fast-paced; the staff manage to cram a lot of songs into the half-hour slot, but if you don't know them there's no assistance or taking it slow – so just clap your hands or sit and listen as it'll soon move onto one you do know.'
Charlotte, mum of Karina

Little Green Frogs
Guildford Spectrum Leisure Complex
Parkway
GU1 1UP
(01483) 443322
(07710) 019455 (Maddy)
(07917) 806065 (Jacqui)
Monday 11.15 am – 12.00 pm

'The usual mix: singing songs (some familiar, some new), plenty of actions,

---

The Little Surrey Songbirds
A wealth of singing pleasure & musical discovery

- Pre-school musical fun for kids aged 3 months and over
- Carefully devised programmes to help nurture musical skills
- Promotes physical and social skills, language and numeracy
- Weekly classes in Guildford held by professional singer/actress

Also available for parties!

Phone 01483 853695
or email surrey@littlesongbirds.com
for details and a free trial
www.littlesongbirds.com

instruments and a bit of marching about, plus parachute play. Bubble chasing and a *'Little Green Frogs'* sticker at the end went down well. No need to book or sign up for a term; just turn up.'
Victoria, mum of Catherine

Little Surrey Songbirds
(01483) 853695 / (0870) 116 4321
(Michele de Casanove)
surrey@littlesongbirds.com
www.littlesongbirds.com

'This is an excellent preschool music class. The classes include singing, percussion and dancing. The teacher, Michele, is excellent at keeping the children involved and makes creative use of toys and props. There is just the right balance of repetition and new material. I've been taking Charlotte since she was four months and it's the highlight of our week.'
Rachel, mum of Charlotte

'Michele has a wonderful singing voice and engages all the children right from the start. The class is great fun and includes action songs and playing a variety of percussion instruments. Michele always includes a couple of soft animal toys to sing about each week, which the children adore. Emily enjoys the classes immensely and has learned lots of new songs. You can either pay for a term or pay-as-you-go each week.'
Angela, mum of Sophie and Emily.

'This music group was enjoyed by our children from birth to age three and they thoroughly enjoyed the mixture of singing, dancing and playing instruments. It is run by Michele, a professional singer and actress, who has a great rapport with the children.'
Rachel, mum of Amy, Thomas and Ella

The Music Box
(01483) 203165 / 202740
judith@yehudimenuhinschool.co.uk
www.yehudimenuhinschool.co.uk/3_outreach.asp
Venues in Albury and Cobham. Call for details

'These music classes are run in association with the *Yehudi Menuhin School of Music* and are for one to four-year-olds. Ella goes to the Albury class and absolutely loves it. The classes are 30 minutes long and run during term-times. Pre-booking is essential. Each week there is a theme and a different musical instrument. Jane runs the Albury class and her calm and gentle manner has the children captivated. It is a definite highlight of our week.'
Lynn, mum of Ella

Music with Mummy
(01483) 533268
jenny.charles1@ntlworld.com
www.musicwithmummy.co.uk
Venues throughout Surrey. See website for details

'Shortly after we moved to Guildford, I did the rounds of toddler music sample classes, and dismissed all of them until we discovered *'Music with Mummy'*.

Things to Do

We loved it. Gentle, home-based, and with the perfect balance of listening and participating, it was an excellent introduction for Victoria to both music, and a group activity environment. It was just as rewarding for me: I loved getting to know other mothers and children in a fun, supportive and creative atmosphere, and I was distraught when Victoria's busy playgroup schedule finally necessitated giving up music class! She started classes when she was ten months old, and finished when she was three, which is the upper age limit the course is designed for.'
Kris, mum of Olivia and Victoria

'*Music with Mummy*' is a gentle introduction to music and rhythm for preschool children. Each half term there is a theme that recurs every week, so by the end of the term the children (and mums) have a sense of anticipation. I take Louis to Jenny's class in Guildford, and he bounces across the room when it's his turn to 'say hello', and he loves playing the instruments – especially the drum! At home, I often hear him singing the songs, of which there is a good mix of traditional known nursery rhymes and original songs. Very reasonably priced.'
Emma, mum of Charlotte and Louis

Zebedee's Music
(0870) 7502861
Classes in Guildford, Godalming and Wonersh

'All three of my children have loved this music group. It lasts for 35 minutes and is full of interactive songs for both child and parent! It is a great time to spend with your child and is an opportunity for them to really join in and have fun. There are band sacks full of interesting instruments, hand puppets and cuddly toys. My one-year-old adores the drum – both for making a noise and for using the drumstick as a teether! Suitable from six months onwards and the groups are tailored to the relevant age as much as possible.'
Rebecca, mum of Isabelle, Aimee and Robyn

Sing a Song of Sixpence
St Albans Church Hall
Oak Hill
Wood Street Village
GU3 3ES
(01483) 870939 (Michaela Kelly)
michaela@singasongofsixpence.co.uk
www.singasongofsixpence.co.uk
Term-time: Tuesday 9.15 – 10.15 am; 10.30 – 11.30 am
[£4.00 per family includes 30 minutes singing followed by playtime with drinks and snacks.]

'A pay-as-you-go singing class for the under-fours. Classes are fun and use simple props and instruments to complement every song. They are very popular, mainly as a direct result of the teacher's calm, friendly and fun approach. The singing lasts approximately 30 minutes, followed by a well earned coffee break afterwards.'
Jo, mum of Oliver and Jake

Things to Do

Come and join in the fun - sing, dance, learn and be inspired at

'ZEBEDEE'S MUSIC'

- Term time classes
- Classes tailored for individual age groups: 6 Months - 4 Years
- Wide range of children's percussion instruments
- Exciting props, puppets and Toys

Zebedee's Music also helps in many other areas of your child learning and development

Zebedee's Music also does children's Music Parties!

Classes in Guildford, Godalming & Wonersh

For more information and a FREE Please call us on 0870 750 2861

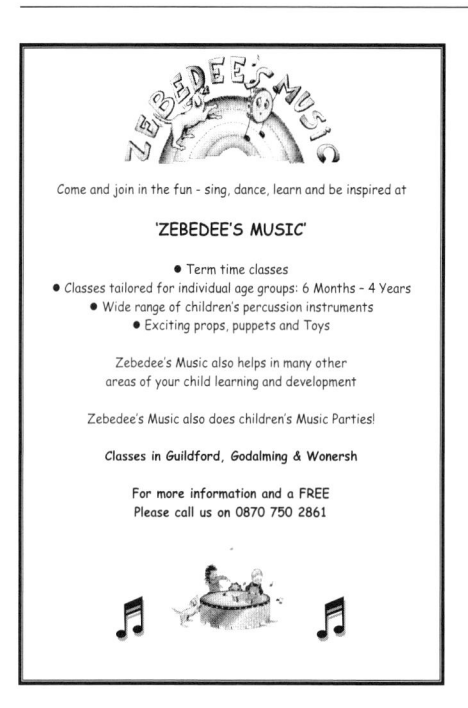

'If you're looking for a friendly informal song group for your baby (no age limit but we've found six months to three years gets the most enjoyment) then give Michaela's *Sing a Song of Sixpence* a visit. For 30 minutes you'll all be singing silly songs with bells, rattles and animals, followed by a half hour play session with refreshments. Michaela is great with the kids and ensures that they are all included, whether they are marching round the room or sitting on mum's lap. You'll be singing songs all week – we haven't missed a session for two and a half years! The sessions can get quite busy so turn up early to avoid disappointment.'

Jenny, mum of Imogen and Harrison

Signing

Sing and Sign
Emmanuel Church Hall
Stoughton
GU2 9SJ
(01252) 641815
singandsignfarnham@hotmail.co.uk
www.singandsign.co.uk
Classes in Godalming, Guildford, Farnham and Fleet

'Although most of the songs are exclusive to *Sing and Sign* you really pick them up very quickly and they are a great way of remembering the signs. You will mix with similar age children and stay together as a group so can really get to know other parents and children. Emmanuel Church has a great coffee/snack bar for afterwards, and it's very child/baby friendly.'
Avril, mum of Scarlett

'Qualified instructors teach babies and parents various signs to avoid frustration in baby when the word itself has not been learned. Signs are learned through music and rhyme. *Sing and*

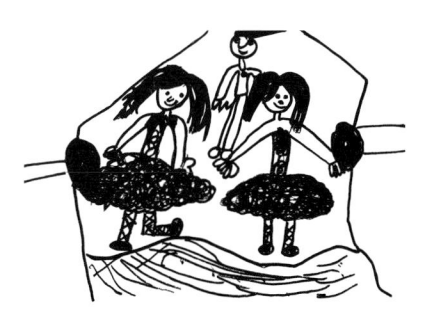

49

Sign is a multi-venue business to suit anyone in and around Guildford and is on various days during the week. There are two stages and you are encouraged to complete a stage twice to cement learning. A stage costs £55.00 and sessions are half an hour. You receive handouts at the end of each session and DVDs or videos are available. An excellent way to encourage communication, and in addition babies enjoy the music and singing.'
Anna, mum of Logan

Time to Sign
(01420) 488339 / (07950) 026542 (Alison Williams)
info@timetosign.co.uk
www.timetosign.co.uk
Classes held in Liphook or privately

'Thomas and I have just finished the 'Progress Course' taught by Alison Williams, and have really enjoyed both it, and the 'Beginners Course' before it. Alison's style makes her very easy to watch and memorable. The classes covered different baby-friendly topics each week (e.g. eating, animals), and included songs and stories. The babies were especially taken with the songs. *Time to Sign* has public courses held in Liphook, but also offers to run them in your own home. A group of us got together and arranged for Alison to give both six week courses at one of our houses in Guildford. At ten months Thomas hasn't started signing back to me yet, but I'm optimistic, as he's very entertained when I sign and sign the songs to him. I'm hoping that the wide vocabulary Alison has given us should help him let me know what he wants before he's talking.'
Fiona, mum of Thomas

Tiny Talk
St Pius Roman Catholic Church Hall
Lauston Close (off Horseshoe Lane East)
Merrow
GU1 2TS
(0870) 242 4898
(07990) 722884 (Louise Derry)
louisede@tinytalk.co.uk
info@tinytalk.co.uk
www.tinytalk.co.uk
Friday 10.00 – 11.00; 11.15 – 12.15
£50.00 for a 12-week course / £4.50 per hour

'*Tiny Talk* is a baby signing organisation, originally started in Guildford, but now running classes all over the UK, and also some classes in Ireland and Australia. The hour-long class consists of 30 minutes learning signs and incorporating signs into songs. The second half of the class is time for babies to play and mums to drink coffee and have a chat.

The theory is that learning signs will assist your child with language acquisition and help with those sticky situations when you really don't understand what your toddler is trying to say to you. Although babies usually won't start signing until they are around 12 months old, the classes can be enjoyed by much younger babies; my 16-month-old has been going to the classes since he was about six months old.

Things to Do

THE MUSIC BOX
EARLY LEARNING THROUGH MUSIC

Classes for 1-4 year olds in Albury and Cobham run by professional musicians

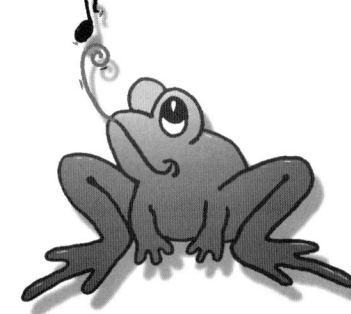

in association with The Yehudi Menuhin School of Music

FOR BOOKING AND MORE INFORMATION, PLEASE CALL
01483 203165   OR   07891 959985

'I have been less than conscientious about signing with my son at home, so I can't say that signing has been a huge success for us. However, we have really enjoyed the classes and have learned lots of new songs (and been reminded of some old favourites too).'
Louise, mum of James

Cinema and Theatre

Children's Theatre
The Mill Studio
Yvonne Arnaud Theatre
Millbrook
GU1 3UX
(01483) 440000
yat@yvonne-arnaud.co.uk
www.yvonne-arnaud.co.uk

'Several Saturdays a month, the *Mill Studio*, next to the main *Yvonne Arnaud Theatre* runs great children's theatre shows. Check out the website for age suitability [and times and prices] before you book, but we have been taking our son there from the age of two and he has always thoroughly enjoyed himself. The shows last about 45 minutes and we've always been amazed at the skill of the actors in keeping a theatre full of toddlers amused and seated for the duration. It's all quite relaxed and no-one minds if your child needs to go to the toilet halfway through! The café in the *Yvonne Arnaud Theatre* is a great place for a drink and a snack afterwards too.
Julie, mum of Ben and Katie

Things to Do

Little Sparks
The Electric Theatre
Onslow Street
GU1 4SZ
(01483) 444789 / (07949) 821567 (Geoff)
www.guildford.gov.uk
Saturday 11.00 am
£4.00 per child. Adults and babies are free

'This is an opportunity to keep the little ones (under-fives) occupied with an hour of entertainment at the weekend. *Little Sparks* is hosted by a couple, who sing songs, tell stories and provide other entertaining activities. Ideal for a morning activity combined with the Saturday market shop!'
Cathi, mum of Ben and Ella

'This drop-in music session is great fun, and perfect to escape to with your little one(s) while your other half goes shopping in town. Geoff and Sue are natural with kids, and classes seem to remain small enough to feel personal and cosy.'
Paige, mum of Miranda and Leo

Odeon Kids Club
Odeon Guildford
Bedford Road
GU1 4SJ
(0871) 22 44 007 (Filmline)
www.odeon.co.uk
Saturday and Sunday 11.00 (check first, times may vary).
[For every child the adult is free. Children £2.50 or meal deal £4.50 including ticket, drink, popcorn, and packet of sweets. ODEON Kids also runs every weekend throughout school holiday periods, with the exception of bank holiday weekends.]

'This has got to be one of the best value weekend activities for kids. Sooo much cheaper than going to the cinema any other time. You have to watch the designated *Odeon Kids* film for that week. These are a recent kids film or modern classic; they are published a couple of months ahead, (see website or get a leaflet from the foyer), then put the ones you want to see in your diary. These are starting to get more popular so might be worthwhile to book in advance. Make sure you know what the film will be and make it clear to the salesperson that it is the *Kids Club* at £2.50, (not all the staff are all aware of this great offer, or of the meal deal – and this includes staff at the food kiosks!) Get a child booster seat where you hand in your ticket (big plastic square that fits over seat so child can see and keeps seat from flipping up). Enjoy!'
Helen, mum of Dominic and Laura

Odeon Newbies (parent and baby screenings)
Odeon Guildford
Bedford Road
GU1 4SJ
(0871) 22 44 007 (Filmline)
www.odeon.co.uk
[Screenings are on weekday mornings, check in advance for times and films. Tickets are priced as normal with babies going for free. *Odeon Newbies* is

The Electric Theatre
Guildford

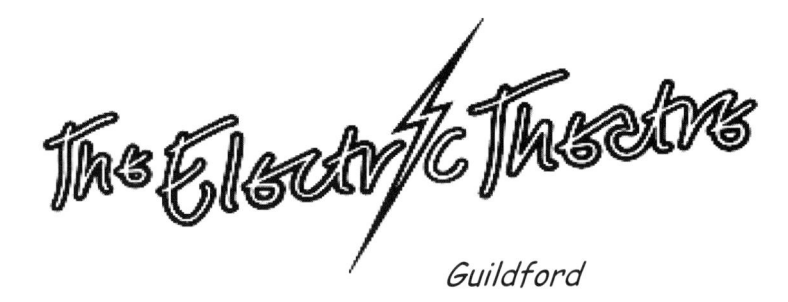

Welcomes you and your family

- You'll find us at the bottom of Guildford's North Street – just cross over from the Friary Centre, walk along the river or take the subway beside Woolworths!

- Every Saturday we have a children's show for the under 5s in our Farley Room upstairs. 'Little Sparks' provide a 40 minute show with music, stories, puppets, games and songs. For more details look on our website! For older children we have regular drama workshops and shows.

- In our airy and relaxing Café Bar you can sit outside or inside and enjoy anything from a cake and coffee to a delicious meal. Why not call to book a table on 01483 444 786?

- We're easy to access with ramped access for pushchairs, level floors, a buggy park, high chairs and baby change facilities

To find out more please ring Box Office on 01483 444789 or check the website www.electrictheatre.co.uk

especially for parents with new babies. Watch current film releases with your baby. Parents are encouraged to bring their babies along to the screening, so there is no need to worry about your little one making any noise. The films are slightly quieter and the lights are raised more than usual, creating a more calming environment. All films will be certificate 12A or lower.]

'Good when your baby's very young and just dozes/feeds through the film. A great idea and enjoyable on your own or with friends.'
Victoria, mum of Catherine

Baby Massage/Baby Yoga

We all know how exhausting those first few weeks/months/years can be! Time to relax seems something of the past but with baby massage it doesn't have to be. Having an hour each week in those early months can be a haven for learning how to massage our babies safely and effectively. Not only is it therapeutic for them it is lovely for mums too.

Baby Massage Teacher and Reflexologist – Monique Harrison
Sundials
1 Beech Lane
GU2 4ES
(01483) 537788

'Monique held a baby massage class for our postnatal group of new dads and four-month-old babies. The dads (and apparently the babies) enjoyed it, and it certainly gave the dads more confidence in handling their babies. It was quite down to earth and the course was more than just massage.'
Victoria, mum of Catherine

'I haven't used Monique for baby massage, but she's been fantastic for me! She takes clients at *Neal's Yard* or at home, and being so into babies she is always happy to have a little one amusing itself in the corner of the room while you submit to the joys of being pummelled. She will even wipe their noses and retrieve tossed toys, or let you breastfeed while she does your feet! Highly recommended.'
Paige, mum of Miranda and Leo

Willow Sanctuary
(antenatal, postnatal, general yoga and baby massage)
Watts Cottage
Jacobs Well
GU4 7PP
(01483) 824838
www.yoga-guildford.com
mich_morrow@hotmail.com

'Michelle holds classes in a purpose-built cabin in the grounds of her home, and provides all the equipment (mats, blankets and cushions) needed. The groups are small with some mums returning after

antenatal classes (like me), and some who were completely new. The time is split equally to focus on both you as an individual, and you with baby. I always found this to be a peaceful time to be with my daughter and (baby permitting) to relax and bond (away from the mania of laundry and dirty dishes at home). As you would expect there would always be at least one baby who either didn't want to participate or insisted on being fed all the way through the session, but the atmosphere was so relaxed this would never cause a problem as we all knew it would probably be us the following week!'
Sandra, mum of Eloise

Sarah Church
Greenfields Yoga Centre
Glaziers Lane
Normandy
GU3 2DQ
(07816) 534554
sarah@yoga-surrey.co.uk
www.yoga-surrey.co.uk

'This was a thoroughly enjoyable postnatal yoga course both for babies and mums. The session involved relaxation and stretching exercises for the mums as well as fun exercises and songs for the babies. There were also two baby massage classes included within the ten sessions. The classes were a great way of meeting other people. My daughter very much enjoyed all the activity and certainly slept very well after each class!'
Dimitra, mum of Electra

Dance classes

Boogie Babies
Sports Centre
University of Surrey
(01483) 689201
www.unisport.co.uk
Term-time Monday 10.00 – 11.00 (no need to book in advance, just turn up.) [See website for details of many other activities for school-age kids. Sessions include songs, movement activities, parachute play for up to five-year-olds]

'*Boogie Babies* is a great way to start your week. It's on a Monday morning in the sports hall on campus. The class is taken by Laura, who is enthusiastic and full of energy. The music is great, and liked by all. There is a good mix of familiar and new activities, and plenty of space to let the little ones run around. The class always ends with a ride on a big cloth parachute which is pulled round by the adults.'
Liz, mum of Thomas

Godalming School of Dance
Culmer Croft
Petworth Road
Wormley
GU8 5SW
(01428) 682175 (Carys Ritchie)
(01483) 416055 (Sandra Avenell)
Classes held in Guildford, Godalming and Ash

'*Godalming School of Dance* has a really good reputation for teaching dance, which was why I chose it. Charlotte goes to Mrs

Raymond's ballet class in Onslow Village, and absolutely loves it. She is constantly showing me 'good' and 'naughty' toes, curtseys, and general spins, skips and dances that she has learned. It is the favourite of all her activities, and I think she'll be going for a long while yet.

Children start at the age of three, and classes start with ballet, then when children reach the age of five they can do modern jazz and tap. Classes are parent-free, but parents are invited to watch on the last day of term. All teachers are qualified and registered with the Royal Academy of Dance (RAD) and the Imperial Society of Teachers of Dance (ISTD).

Exam work starts at the age of six. Ballet exams are through the RAD and modern and tap through the ISTD.'
Emma, mum of Charlotte and Louis

Italia Conti Arts Centre
221 Epsom Road
Merrow
GU1 2RE
(01483) 568070 / 565967
www.italia-conti.co.uk

'We have been going for almost two years. My daughter, who is now four, loves it. She does both ballet and tap classes and has taken part in one show. The teachers are very nice and I enjoy having a coffee and chat to the other mums in the lounge. The front of the school has a nice shop where you can buy the outfits, shoes and many lovely presents.'
Thora, mum of Freyja

Patricia Ellis School of Dancing
6 Wheeler Street
Witley
GU8 5LX
(01428) 682896
Classes held in Onslow Village, Guildford and Witley

'My three-year-old daughter has just completed her first term of ballet lessons here, and she absolutely loves it. The ballet classes are on Mondays and the first class is for two and a half to four-year-olds. The lessons are half an hour in length and while they aren't too serious, it is mostly about fun, there is a certain amount of discipline that they all seem to respond well to.'
Katherine, mum of Holly and Hazel

Linda Ryder
74 Agraria Road
GU2 4LG
(01483) 564517
linda.ryder@lineone.net

'Emily (four) has been eagerly attending Linda's ballet classes for 18 months now and James (three) has just started. From the very beginning Emily has absolutely loved it. She shows us her 'tickly feet' and 'tidy feet' and regales us with wonderful stories of castles, knights, princesses, swaying trees and funny monsters. Linda is such a creative and gentle person that I can think of no better introduction to the world of ballet. She has converted her living room into a dance studio, so her home environment creates a relaxed and informal setting. The children can wear

whatever they want, although most of the girls opt for the full ballet regalia and the boys tend to wear shorts and T-shirts. The children usually attend without their parents, although parents and siblings are proudly invited to watch the last class of each term. Linda teaches ballet from three years old until adulthood. The children's classes are held on Saturday mornings for 40 minutes and in small groups of no more than nine. They are very reasonably priced and worth every penny!'
Cally, mum of Emily and James

Planet Dance
16A Bartholomew Close
Haslemere
GU27 1EN
(07940) 500510 (Sam Punter)
(07967) 397379 (Becky Moore-Morris)
Classes held in Guildford, Godalming and Liphook

'It's really nice to find a pay-as-you-go dance class that's a bit different. Sam and Becky are IDTA trained, and specialise in freestyle modern dance, from street jazz to rock 'n' roll. They teach children from as young as two and a half up to young-at-heart adults (like me). What's even more fun, is that every 18 months *Planet Dance* holds a dance show where all participants of all classes have the opportunity to get up on stage (usually at *Princes Theatre*, Aldershot) and 'strut their stuff' for family and friends – usually to an audience of about 600! In-between show rehearsals you can take exams, thereby continuously improving your technique. This year (2007) Charlotte and I were both in a dance show, which was really exciting and such a lovely thing to do together, and next time I hope Louis will be there too – he's just about old enough to join now!
Emma, mum of Charlotte and Louis

Art Activities

For all those budding artists this section is for you. Even if you lack artistic talent there is nothing quite like sitting down with a paint brush and going wild, nothing more hypnotic than playing with modelling clay, and nothing more rewarding than seeing the final product after all your 'hard' work – the children love it too! This section details a number of venues that encourage you to do all these and more, and with careful supervision there are people on hand to guide you with ideas when your artistic innovation dries up!

The 06 Pottery Café
60 High Street
Godalming
GU7 1DU
(01483) 527275

'About six weeks before Christmas we made a booking for five of us and our six month old babies, buggies etc. to go along and make up some baby prints for gifts for the family. The table was all laid

Things to Do

out and the guys inside were exceptional at helping us to set up and even helped with holding babies. They served great coffee, and we ordered pizza from down the road and ate after our prints were done. A really good way to spend a morning or afternoon, and outstanding service!'
Avril, mum of Scarlett

'A wonderful pottery café to create once-in-a-lifetime baby footprint/handprint memories. The manager is exceptionally helpful, polite and knowledgeable. The venue is small but manages to fit buggies and babies well. The manager will order and deliver lunch from the nearby pizza place if requested. A large assortment of ceramics can be purchased and painted, from plates and bowls, to Christmas ornaments and flower pots. For creative people there is a large array of various painting implements. You need to wait a week for glazing before collecting. A baby-changing mat is available and a wide selection of beverages can be bought. Breastfeeding is encouraged. The manager and his assistant do a fantastic, confident job of helping you imprint your baby's hands or feet into your chosen ceramic and create a wonderful memory that will last forever.'
Anna, mum of Logan

Firing Earth
82 Smithbrook Kilns
A281 Horsham Road
Cranleigh
GU6 8JJ
(01483) 268788
www.firingearth.co.uk

'We had a group of six adults and six children, and it was a fun way to spend a morning. You can pre-book for groups or turn up individually. You choose from the display which pieces of crockery you would like to decorate and then get painting! You leave them to be fired, and then pick them up a week or two later. There are no toilet facilities but you can buy drinks. After the budding artists had finished and feet and hands were all clean we then went to the nearby café for lunch.'
Lynn, mum of Ella

Hands of Clay
Camilla Goldsmith
Anstey House
97 Anstey Road
Alton
GU34 2RL
(01420) 87597
camilla@handsofclay.co.uk

'Camilla from *Hands of Clay* came to join us at our weekly NCT get-together.

GETTING YOU BACK INTO SHAPE

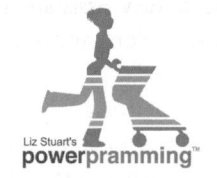

Liz Stuart's
powerpramming™

Classes now running in this area, please contact Clare on 07979 694758 for details.
www.powerpramming.co.uk

She needs a minimum of six people to come out, but you can also visit her studio in Alton if you prefer. You can choose from any combination of baby, sibling or parent handprints and footprints, varying in price from about £12.00 upwards, depending on the size. I opted for my handprint next to my baby's little handprint on one piece of clay and two baby footprints on another, but any combination is possible. They are very quick and simple to do – just press hand and/or foot into a piece of soft, rolled out clay, then Camilla takes them away to be fired in the kiln. A really lovely reminder of just how small your baby was as they grow up.'
Julie, mum of Ben and Katie

Potty Paintbrush
12 Haydon Place (off North Street)
GU1 4LL
(01483) 533218
info@thepottypaintbrush.com
www.thepottypaintbrush.com

'I went with my friend and three under-twos. The shop assistant was very helpful with suggestions for Father's Day designs and helped with footprints and handprints. Along with crockery there was a selection of child-orientated ornaments ready for decoration. We had a double buggy that, although was tight getting into the shop, had plenty of space once inside. No toilet facilities but tea and coffee are available.'
Sarah, mother of Benedict and Jolyan

Story Time

We all know the benefits of reading with our children and getting them to enjoy looking at books. Other than taking time-out at home to read with them, you may like to join a few other mums and make it a sociable event.

Guildford Library 'Storytime'
Guildford Library
77 North Street
GU1 4AL
(08456) 009009
libraries@surreycc.gov.uk
www.surreycc.gov.uk
Friday 2.15 pm – 2.45 pm

'I have now been a couple of times to the library with my nearly three-year-old on Friday afternoons, where there is half an hour of stories read by one of the library assistants for free! It is held in the children's section at the back of the ground floor. There are some seats (not many!) and cushions for parent and child to use while listening to the stories. The library assistant reads well and with expression, and the books he chooses work well for the age range of two to five-year-olds. The library offers a great resource for preschoolers to browse and borrow books, with no penalties and a three-week borrowing time. Only downside is you will need to vacate the

Things to Do

library for the toilet, the nearest are the public ones across the road!'
Carolyn, mother of Jessica

Teddies Ten Minutes
All Saints Church
Onslow Village
GU2 7QJ
(01483) 572006
info@allsaintschurchgfd.org.uk
www.allsaintschurchgfd.org.uk
Tuesday 2.00 pm

'*Teddies Ten Minutes* is an informal story time for toddlers and preschool-aged children at *All Saints Church*. It is very informal – the vicar lights a candle for each child present and then reads a story. She is extremely good with children and my toddler loves it.

Afterwards, there are drinks and biscuits for the children and parents, and a chance for the little ones to run around and play hide and seek in the church!'
Liz, mum of Isabelle and Evie

Ante/Postnatal Exercise and Support

Keen to get fit again but not sure where you can take your baby while you have a quick work out, then carry on reading. Guildford *Spectrum* is the main leisure centre in Guildford but there are also some smaller venues that might suit you better. Happy exercising!

Circuit Training
Emmanuel Church Parish Centre
Shepherd's Lane
Stoughton
GU2 9SJ
(01483) 561603 (church office)
[These classes have now moved to Guildford Spectrum park, and are held outdoors on Wednesday evenings]

'These classes are fantastic if you're just venturing back to exercise after having a baby or have older kids and want a fun way of keeping fit. The sessions have a friendly feel, and Chrissi takes care to make sure that everyone can exercise at their own level. The crèche is run each week by Joan and volunteer mums who take it in turns; it's full of toys and books to keep the little ones entertained while you exercise. You can either pay-as-you-go or buy ten sessions at once with a reduction. There's even a chance for a coffee and chat afterwards in the Parish Centre coffee shop.'
Jo, mum of Stanley

'These classes are taught by a qualified midwife 'Chrissi' who is excellent, and whom I found personally helpful in ensuring my technique was appropriate for my postnatal return to a more challenging routine. Classes are always varied to ensure you're not bored, and usually are circuit style routines rather than complicated aerobic moves for those

Things to Do

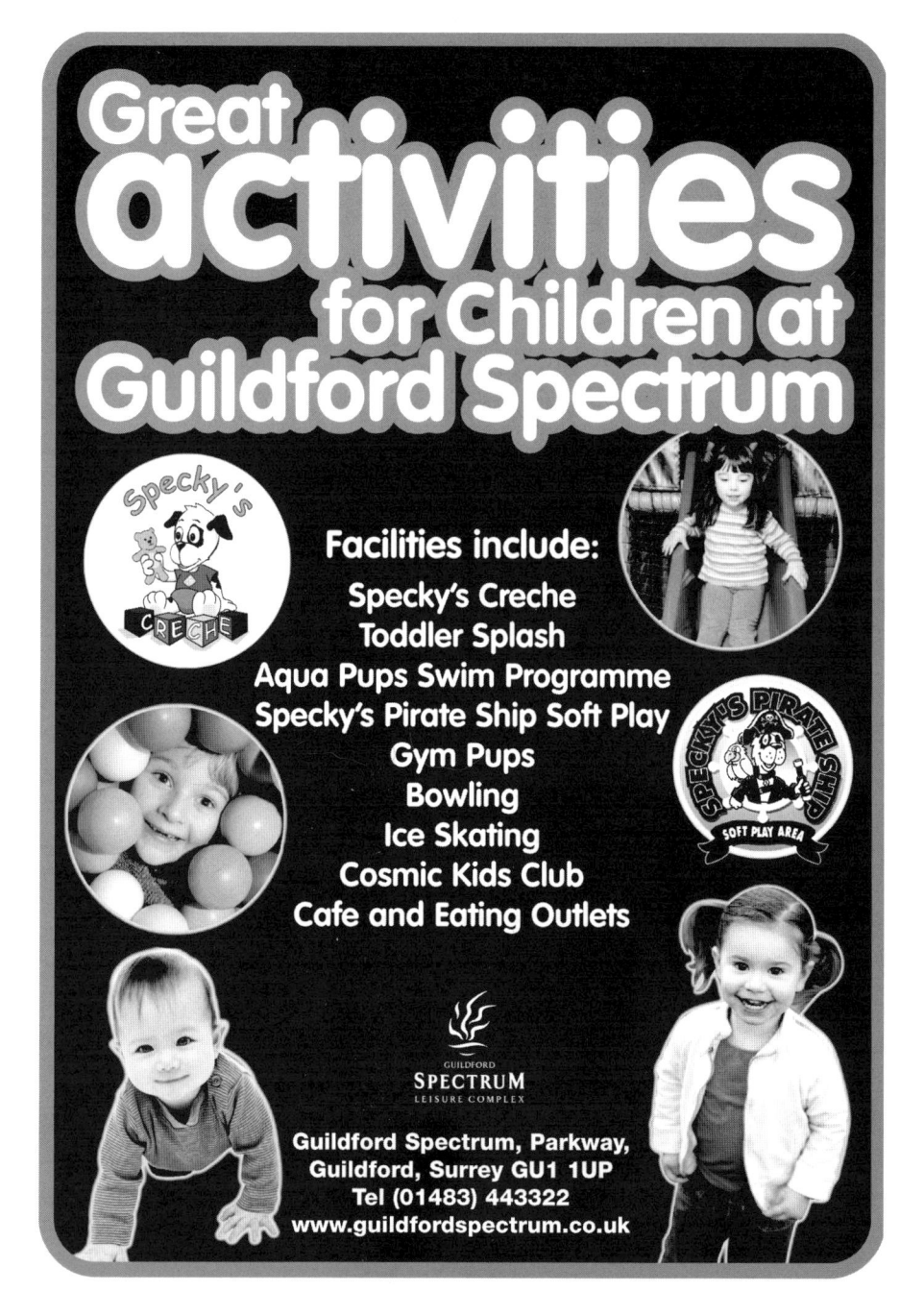

Great activities for Children at Guildford Spectrum

Facilities include:
Specky's Creche
Toddler Splash
Aqua Pups Swim Programme
Specky's Pirate Ship Soft Play
Gym Pups
Bowling
Ice Skating
Cosmic Kids Club
Cafe and Eating Outlets

GUILDFORD
SPECTRUM
LEISURE COMPLEX

Guildford Spectrum, Parkway,
Guildford, Surrey GU1 1UP
Tel (01483) 443322
www.guildfordspectrum.co.uk

Things to Do

PERSONAL FITNESS TRAINER

Pre & Postnatal Fitness
- Weight Loss – Toning – Strength
- Core Conditioning – and much more...
Let me help you look good and feel great!
Call me for a **FREE** consultation

Becky Moore-Morris
(Dip.PT, IIST, AIDTA, ETM)
(07987) 397379

---

less coordinated (particularly after a sleepless night). A crèche is coordinated by the mums and the little one can be watched for a nominal fee.'
Cathi, mum of Ben and Ella

Badminton

*Guildford Spectrum Leisure Complex
Parkway
GU1 1UP
(01483) 443322
www.guildfordspectrum.co.uk*

'Our postnatal group wanted to keep meeting after our courses ended, so we booked out one of the sports halls in the *Spectrum* and played badminton while our babies played, fed or slept on gym mats at the side of the gym.

The booking included having the court set up for us (however need to bring your own racquets and shuttlecocks), and use of the room for an hour or two. I don't remember the cost, but it wasn't much. We played loads of games of badminton while rotating baby-entertaining duties, and breastfed when we needed to.

Often we'd stop for a coffee in the café afterwards too. It was a great way to have a bit of exercise, fun and sociability in those early months.

We only stopped when too many babies had started crawling and thus were interfering with our game!'
Paige, mum of Miranda and Leo

Dunk Your Bump

*Guildford Spectrum Leisure Complex
Parkway
GU1 1UP
(01483) 443322
www.guildfordspectrum.co.uk
Tuesday 11.00 – 11.45 am, Wednesday 8.00 – 8.45 pm*

'These water aerobic classes are run by midwives from the *Royal Surrey County Hospital* and are for pregnant ladies and new mothers; however, when I went on a Tuesday morning I only ever saw pregnant ladies there.

It is a gentle water workout, which is fun, and you even get to do your pelvic floor exercises yet again. It is very good for meeting people especially in your first pregnancy and I made some wonderful friends there.'
Nadine, mum of Noah and Luca

'*Dunk Your Bump* is geared specifically for pregnant mothers and taught by a qualified midwife. Swimming and gentle water aerobics is the best non-impact exercise for your growing shape, and if you are working, Wednesday evening is a good opportunity to squeeze some exercise into your schedule.'
Cathi, mum of Ben and Ella

Post/Antenatal Exercise

(Also held at Guildford Spectrum, see above)
Thursday 11.00 – 12.00

'This class is great for starting to get fit after baby. There is room for prams, so everyone parks their babies at the back of the room or puts them on mats or blankets and the music (mostly) drowns out the screams by the end of the session. The instructor is friendly and the exercises gentle. Best of all is the coffee (and cake if you're feeling naughty) afterwards in the café upstairs, where there are highchairs and room for pushchairs. Usually mums have stopped going by the time baby starts crawling, as it's hard to exercise around them.'
Kelley, mum of Audrey

'This class is fantastic for keeping fit and healthy with a growing baby inside you antenatally, and for easing back into a regular exercise routine postnatally. An hour of gentle aerobics taught by a very enthusiastic and cheerful 'Louise' is enjoyable, babies are welcome and are always found playing to the music and watching mum making 'funny' moves!'
Cathi, mum of Ben and Ella

Legs, Bums and Tums

(Also held at Guildford Spectrum, see above)
Tuesday 9.45 am and 6.00 pm
Friday 9.45 am

'This class has been taught by a fantastic instructor 'Kerri' for at least three years now and will guarantee results for your postnatal figure. This is an adult-only class, but the crèche can watch little ones from three months old. I found the need to phone ahead with the crèche to avoid disappointment, however, as 'LBT' is most popular with mums and there is often a waiting list.'
Cathi, mum of Ben and Ella

Crèche

(Also at Guildford Spectrum, see above)
Monday to Friday 8.30 am – 1.30 pm

'I have used the crèche here on and off for four years. It is great value at £2.60 for up to two hours. The staff are friendly and welcoming to new children. All children have their own coat peg and you write any special instructions, e.g. dietary needs, snack times etc., up on the white board for all to see. You do need to book a week in advance so some organization on your part is required. There is a good selection of toys available and also sometimes a craft activity.'
Alison, mum of Laura and Daniel

The Herons Swimming and Fitness Centre

Kings Road
Haslemere
GU27 2QA
(01428) 658484
enquiries@theheronsswimandfitnesscentre.co.uk
www.dcleisurecentres.co.uk

'The gym has been recently renovated with state-of-the-art equipment and personal TV screens. Sauna and steam room also

available. There are crèche facilities for children from six weeks to four years.'
Nicki, mum of George and Olivia

The Mother Mentor
Maja Pawinska Sims
(01483) 561711
maja@themothermentor.com
www.themothermentor.com

Maja supports new mums through the intense highs and challenges of the first year of their babies' lives with a one-to-one coaching programme. In 45-minute face-to-face or telephone sessions, she helps you work out the right decisions and action for you, your baby and your family on any area, including expectations of motherhood, being a good enough mother, communication with partners and others, feeding, routines, childcare, and returning to work.

PowerPramming
Clare Davis
(07979) 694758
clare@claredavisfitness.co.uk
www.powerpramming.com
Classes currently running in Woking and Brooklands

'*Powerpramming* is a good way to take the little one for some fresh air with other new mums. This is particularly good if you struggle to leave the house during a dreary, grey winter maternity leave. The instructor is a qualified personal trainer with extra training in antenatal and postnatal exercise.'
Cathi, mum of Ben and Ella

And Finally ...Holiday Activities

Not sure what to do with the little ones during the school holidays? Your regular groups are term-time only? Do not despair, there are still plenty of organised activities out there. Here are a few ideas. Check out the holiday activities run by *Guildford Spectrum* (go in a few weeks before the holidays for a leaflet and pre-book), *Woking Leisure Centre* and the *North Guildford Children's Centre*. Ring first to check times and age limits.

Caterpillar Café
Church of the Holy Spirit
New Inn Lane
Burpham
GU4 7HW
(01483) 571686 (Katie Thomas)
me@katiethomas.co.uk
www.burphamchurch.org.uk
Friday 10.00 – 11.30
[See review under 'Toddler Groups' p20]

Guildford Children's Centre (North Guildford site) – Play and Learn
Hazel Avenue
GU1 1NR
(01483) 566589
admin@guildfordchildrenscentre.surrey.sch.uk
www.guildfordchildrenscentre.sch.uk
Holiday Drop-in *Play and Learn* (up to three years, see main review p18). More

frequent drop-in sessions than during term-time. Try to arrive on time to avoid disappointment as numbers are limited. Note that the Town Centre site holds occasional fun days. during the holidays. Call the North Guildford site for details.

Child-friendly gardens, open daily, with ride-on toys, sandpit, water-play. There is also a room in the centre with drink-making facilities. During holidays gardens are open most days and are for the use of children under-11 and their carers. Access is also limited in numbers.

Guildford Spectrum Leisure Complex
Parkway
GU1 1UP
(01483) 443322
www.guildfordspectrum.co.uk
[Other holiday activities include *Chelsea Soccer School* (four to five years); *Junior Summer Fitness Challenge* (where children have to do and record 20-30 minutes of activities per day in return for rewards); *Learn to Swim* (from beginners); *Parent and Toddler Bounceabout* (18 months to five years); *Specky's Holiday Gympups* (see review below and 'Sporting Activities' p25); *Super Tots* (three to five years); *Tennis Together* (three to five years); *Trampoline* (three to five years). See website for details]

'*Specky's Holiday Gympups* is a fun and lively soft play session, which is aimed at 18 months to four years and provides a range of gym equipment including a bouncy castle, a ball pond, trampoline and play tunnels. Sessions are popular and you have to pre-book. They usually start around 9.30 am and last for an hour. A great option for the holidays.'
Jo, mum to Oliver and Jake

Gym Jams
Normandy Village Hall
Manor Fruit Farm
Glaziers Lane
Normandy
GU3 2DE
(01932) 340379 (Barry or Millie)
info@gym-jams.co.uk
www.gym-jams.co.uk
Wednesday 9.30 – 11.00 am;
11.15 am – 12.45 pm; 1.00 pm – 2.30 pm
Friday 9.30 – 11.30 am
[See review under 'Soft Play' p40 earlier in this chapter]

Gymnastics Factory
Pew Corner
Old Portsmouth Road
GU3 1LP
(01483) 455060
info@gymnasticsfactory.co.uk
www.gymnasticsfactory.co.uk
[See reviews under 'Sporting Activities' p23 and *Services* - 'Parties' p169]

The *Gymnastics Factory* runs holiday sessions with differing themes each week – from improver classes to circus skills, from three hour morning classes (designed for parents to have a morning off) to master classes for those ready to

65

Things to Do

try some advanced skills. Pop in or check out website for details.

Leatherhead & Dorking Gymnastics Club
Leatherhead Leisure Centre car park
Guildford Road
Fetcham
Leatherhead
KT22 9BL
(01372) 377718
[Call for holiday sessions and prices. See also 'Sporting Activities p24]

Rainbow Tots
Knaphill Scout Hall
Waterers Rise
Knaphill
Woking
GU21 2HU
(07803) 600720 (Angela Sanderson)
(07885) 702414 (Hazel Stevens)
info@rainbowtots.com
www.rainbowtots.com
Soft play for under-fives, two-hour session
[Check website first to confirm shorter opening times and holiday dates. Also see main review under 'Soft Play' p41]

Rushmoor Gym
The Gymnastics Centre
Pool Road
Aldershot
GU11 3SN
(01252) 320888
info@rushgym.co.uk (Colin and Bernie Wright)
www.rushgym.co.uk

[See website for holiday Playgym; £1.00 per person; see main entries under 'Gymnastics' p24 and 'Soft Play' p43]

Woking Gymnastics Club
Kingfield Road
Woking
GU22 9AA
(01483) 771426
info@woking-gymnastics.co.uk
www.woking-gymnastics.co.uk
[Courses run for different levels and groups over the holidays. Check out website for more details.]

Woking Leisure Centre
Woking Park,
Kingfield Road,
Woking,
GU22 9BA
(01483) 771122
leisurecentre@woking.gov.uk
www.woking.gov.uk

Woking Leisure Centre runs many holiday activities for children, including *Toddler Splash* and a Wednesday morning playgroup (usually 10.00 am – 12.00 pm). The first hour of playgroup includes bouncy castle and various craft activities, followed by a break for juice and biscuit. The second hour includes soft play shapes and trampolines. There is a parachute and songs at the end. Must pre-book.

[See *Services* for details of other activities open in the holidays including Godalming Toy Library, Mobile Library, Guildford Library…]

3
Places to Visit

Julie Stott, mum of Ben and Katie

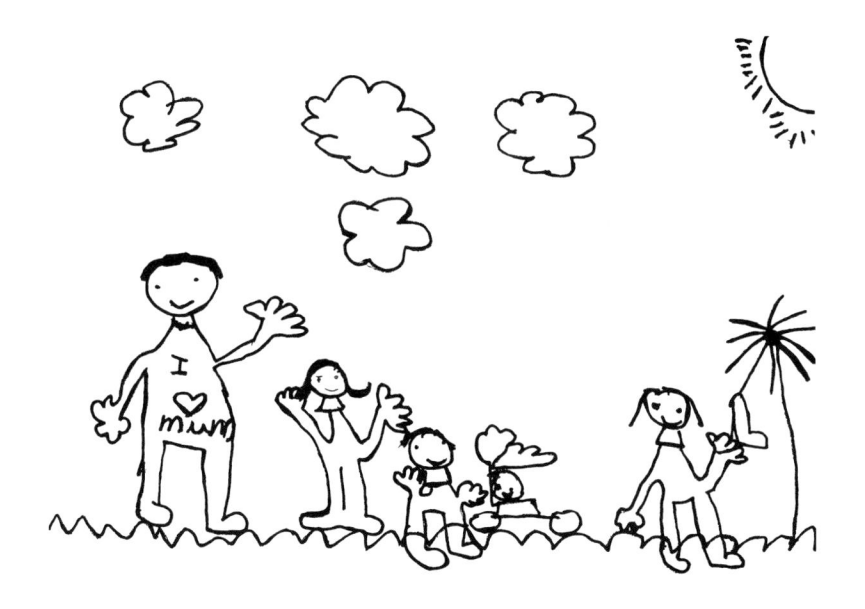

In the early days of parenthood, just getting out of the house can seem like an impossible task. It's not long though, before you start to realise that children are usually much happier (and hence so are you), when they're out and about and you start to wonder just where you can go with a pushchair and an inquisitive child. If you're anything like me, before my children arrived, I have to confess to hardly knowing the very town I lived in. I was always rushing off to work and at weekends went no further than clothes shopping, the pub or my local Indian restaurant – none of which I later came to realise would work well with children!

So what do children enjoy? Well, judging by the huge number and variety of ideas that parents sent into us, there is no shortage of fun, interesting, educational and exciting places to visit in our area. The suitability of each will depend on the age of your child and how adventurous you are feeling, but everything from the joy of seeing little faces light up when you take them to feed the ducks, to a full-blown day out at a theme park is covered here. I've

Places to Visit

really enjoyed trying out some of the recommendations from this chapter and I hope there's plenty for you to enjoy too.

[Guildford Borough Council (*www.guildford.gov.uk/GuildfordWeb/Tourism/Children*) has a page on its website dedicated to places to go for children, with direct links to other fun sites, most of which are included in this book, but it is worth a look if you want a brief snapshot of ideas.]

Farms

Bocketts Farm
Young Street
Fetcham
Leatherhead
KT22 9BS
(01372) 363764
www.bockettsfarm.co.uk

'This is a favourite with us. There are lots of farm animals to see and a pet area too. The outdoor play area has a wide variety of activities for toddlers and older children, including playgrounds, sandpits with diggers, playhouses, trampolines and mini-pedal and electric ride-on tractors. The indoor soft play with large 'Astroslide' is great for children of all ages and especially the dads! There is also a tractor ride (extra cost), which takes you on a mini tour of the farm. The Old Barn is a good tearoom and is well stocked with high chairs and also caters for children's parties.'
Lisa, mum of Thomas

'A great day out catering for all ages with plenty to see and do, from animal petting sessions, to soft play, and many farm animals to see. Under twos are free, but parents currently cost £6.40. Extra costs include animal food, face painting, and tractor and pony rides. Plenty of outside space and play activities but if it rains it can become crowded inside. A popular place for school holidays and weekends.'
Jo, mum of Matthew

'This is a fantastic place, with a wide range of animals, most of which you can feed. You can also watch pig racing and go on tractor and pony rides. If that is not enough, there are fantastic playgrounds outside (including sandpits, trampolines and a giant bouncy air pillow) and two large soft play areas inside. The restaurant is good, but is crowded on busy days. An alternative is to take a picnic as there are lots of picnic tables around the farm.'
Louise, mum of Joseph and Emilia

'Great fun for all the family. Lots of different playgrounds for kids from toddlers to juniors. Go at Easter for baby animals. Good food there, or take a picnic. Lots of walking, so take a buggy for little ones.'
Charlotte, mum of Noah

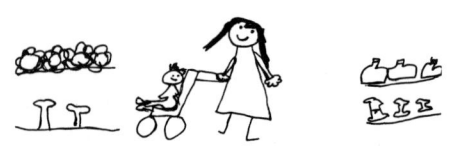

Places to Visit

Burpham Court Farm Park
Clay Lane
Jacobs Well
GU4 7NA
(01483) 576089
www.burphamcourtfarm.com

'Although not quite so well developed as some of the other farms around the area, this is still a great place for real hands-on animal experience. You can purchase bags of food for the sheep, goats, chickens and llamas and watch them compete for your handfuls. There are also often baby guinea pigs to look at and older ones to hold. There are a number of ride-on toys, a big sandpit and an elderly tractor, which is a major draw for young boys.

The highlight of the day is animal feeding time, at about 3.30 pm. All the children help get the feeds ready, collect eggs from the hen houses, and help lock up the goats, llamas and ponies for the night. You can buy limited refreshments. The toilets are basic but clean and there's always soap and anti-bacterial handwash available.'
Sally, mum of James

Fishers Farm Park
Newpound Lane
Wisborough Green
RH14 0EG
(01403) 700063
www.fishersfarmpark.co.uk

'*Fisher's Farm* is about 40 minutes from Guildford, but well worth the drive. The admission price includes all the activities so there are no hidden extras. There's the usual selection of animals and the opportunity for animal handling.

There are several indoor soft play areas next to the café so you can eat or drink while the children play, and a massive outdoor play area with activities for all ages. These include trampolines, a climbing wall, merry-go-rounds, swing boats, climbing frames, big slides, little spinning boats etc. Quad biking is also available for children over the age of eight and in the summer there are [quite deep] paddling pools so it's worth taking swimming things.

There are usually seasonal shows and activities available as well as 'train', tractor, pony and combine harvester rides. You can easily spend the whole day there if you want to make the most of your entrance fee. The café is reasonable; it has the usual child-friendly fare, and is all clean and well presented.'
Bridget, mum of Jessie and Luke

'Huge, award-winning play park and farm, where the family can spend the whole day. There will be something to entertain all your children, irrespective of age. They can jump around on large trampolines, take a ride on the top of a combine harvester, get inside the pens of the animals [goats, sheep, pigs etc] to stroke them, clamber around in the soft play areas, ride the mini-electric-tractors, climb the large roped climbing frame, and then collapse in the restaurant. A lovely day out.'
Sonya, mum of Eleanor and Charles

Places to Visit

Godstone Farm
Tilburstow Hill Road
Godstone
RH9 8LX
(01883) 742546
havefun@godstonefarm.co.uk
www.godstonefarm.co.uk

'Our four-year-old nephew had a whale of a time the day we took him to Godstone Farm. The children's farm had a good variety of animals and birds, and was well laid out. The play facilities were excellent too, with ride-on trucks, slides, karts, adventure playgrounds and sandpits. Around the edge of this area there were well-spaced picnic tables and benches, so it was an ideal place to finish the visit. The farm and play areas all appeared well maintained and the toilets reasonably clean. There is a play barn and tearoom at the farm, although we didn't use either on our visit. Godstone Farm also hosts children's parties, and there are details of the party package on the website.'
Fiona, mum of Thomas

Horton Park Children's Farm
Horton Lane
Epsom
KT19 8PT
(01372) 743984
childrensfarm@hortonpark.co.uk
www.hortonpark.co.uk

'Horton Park Farm is worth the 30 minute trek. There is a selection of farm animals, with large rabbit pens, which the kids can enter to stroke the rabbits. There is also a selection of play areas including bikes, tractors and cars, an undercover sandpit, an undercover climbing wall (suitable for over twos) and slides for all ages. One of the two large play areas has boats and castles to explore and slide down and roam, and the other is mostly for older children. The cost is £5.95 per child (over two) with one adult free per paying child. Extra adults are £5.95 each. There is a play barn with a large soft play area, which is 80p extra. There is a café in the play barn and another in the park itself serving reasonably-priced pastries, coffee and children's packed lunches. There are also many places to have a picnic should you want to take your own. *Horton Park* also does birthday parties.'
Maggie, mum of Alice and Katy

'This farm has a large indoor soft play area, animals, tractor rides and large outdoor play areas. It is good value, especially if you arrange a large group outing. Car parking is no problem.'
Rachel, mum of Amy, Thomas and Ella

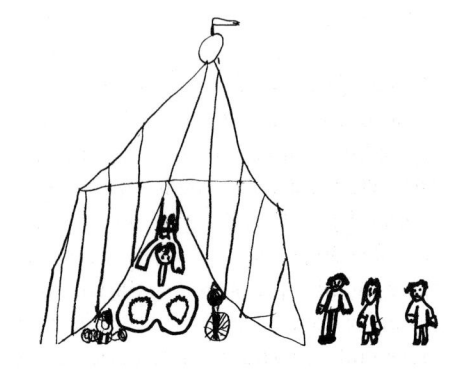

Aquariums, Bird Parks and Zoos

Blue Reef Aquarium
Clarence Esplanade
Southsea
PO5 3PB
(023) 92875222
info@bluereefaquarium.co.uk
www.bluereefaquarium.co.uk/portsmouth.htm

'About one hour's drive from Guildford, this aquarium is the perfect size for toddlers to look around. Lots of colourful fish, a ray 'petting' pool and some otters – just enough to keep them excited, but not too much for little legs. The aquarium café is right on the harbour front, so it's a great place to watch the ferries and boats coming and going after your visit'
Julie, mum of Ben and Katie

Beale Park
Lower Basildon
Reading
RG8 9NH
(0870) 7777160
www.bealepark.co.uk

'This is a little bit of a trek but worth it. It has a good mixture of animals (flamingos, exotic birds, lemurs, monkeys, meerkats, owls etc.) Fab play areas including a special *Little Tikes* 'village' outside and soft play area inside. There is a sandpit, three paddling pools open in the summer, a 'Roplay' rope adventure playground for older children and a water park with a folly that was filled with boat and plane models. The highlight for our train-mad boy was the miniature steam railway. You get one free ride in the cost of the entrance ticket, further rides cost £1.00 each but were absolutely worth every penny. Lots of places to picnic but there is also a café with reasonable food if you fancy a break from preparing food. It currently costs £6.00 off-peak and £8.00 peak time for an adult, and £5.50 for over-twos.'
Jacqui, Mum of Harry and Megan

Birdworld and Underwater World
Holt Pound
Farnham
GU10 4LD
(01420) 22838 (24 hr info); (01420) 22140 (enquiries)
www.birdworld.co.uk

'*Birdworld* is a great day out with babies and toddlers. An annual pass is worthwhile if you plan on visiting more than once although children under three are free. It is a really large enclosed safe environment where toddlers can wander around freely and see all the birds and animals. My two boys just love the little Jenny Wren Farm at the end with lots of animals, the small play area for two to six-year-olds and the red and blue tractors to sit on! Lots of birds to see on the way to the farm with scheduled feeding of the penguins to enjoy. There is a large restaurant at the main entrance, which serves meals until 5.00 pm in the summer and lots of picnic areas and playgrounds. *Underwater World,* situated at the main

entrance, is indoors so good on rainy days with lots of brightly coloured fish to see.'
Marguerite, mum of David and Dylan

'This is a great day out for parents with small children. The park is flat, well-landscaped, and safe for toddlers to roam. The enclosures are all well kept and there is a wide variety of birds and wildlife to see. There is a farm park at the end where the children can handle small animals like rabbits and guinea pigs. There are plenty of places along the way to stop for a snack or you can take a picnic. There is also a play area if the wildlife gets a bit too much!'
Alison, mum of Laura and Daniel

'This is a great place to take children as there is something for everyone. As well as all the birds (including penguins that you can watch being fed) there is a farm with a petting area, tractors to play on, and a small playground. There is also a small aquarium with 'Nemo' and some caiman (like crocodiles).'
Louise, mum of Joseph and Emilia

Drusillas Zoo Park
Alfriston
BN26 5QS
(01323) 874100
info@drusillas.co.uk
www.drusillas.co.uk

'A fabulous children's zoo approximately one and half hour's drive from Guildford. *Drusillas* has a good variety of small animals combined with excellent play facilities suitable for toddlers – it has its own toddler village, and there's a climbing wall and adventure playground suitable for up to 12-year-olds. There is a paddling pool open during the summer and a *Thomas the Tank Engine* mini train. The park has a good choice of eating places and picnic areas with numerous baby-changing facilities. All in all, a great day out.'
Jo, mum of Oliver and Jake

Howletts Wild Animal Park
Bekesbourne
Near Canterbury
CT4 5EL
(0870) 7504647
info@howletts.net
www.totallywild.net/howletts

'This takes about an hour and a half to get to, but it's worth it. *Howletts* has a large gorilla enclosure (there are usually some babies to watch playing) and most other animals you expect. The zoo is not too big so young children can cope with the walking, although it is all pushchair friendly. There are playgrounds too.'
Louise, mum of Joseph and Emilia

London Aquarium
County Hall
Westminster Bridge Road
SE1 7PB
(020) 7967 8000
www.londonaquarium.co.uk

'Located on the South Bank next to the *London Eye*, the Aquarium, combined with the train trip in, makes for a great day out. Both my children were mesmerised by the close-up encounters with sharks and stingrays, which can be observed via two large tanks situated over three floors of the aquarium. There are plenty of smaller tanks to view the fish, and a colouring area to keep little ones occupied.

There are excellent baby-changing facilities on each floor. I would advise pre-booking and getting there when it opens, as it can get busy. As the café is basic and pricey, a picnic is advised, which can always be enjoyed on the South Bank, where there is always plenty going on.'
Jo, mum of Oliver and Jake

Marwell Zoological Park
Colden Common
Winchester
SO21 1JH
(01962) 777407
marwell@marwell.org.uk
www.marwell.org.uk

'We went on a cold February day and took a picnic. Great place for a day out; if you go more than three times a year and live near enough, do consider an annual pass.

There are lots of large and small animals to see and the fences often have glass panels so you don't have to hold your little one up to see the animals over the top! There also is a good play area with wooden climbing frames and swings. It was a bit muddy when we were there, so we were glad we had wellies with us.

There is also a free tractor train to transport little ones (and adults) to or from the entrance (with a dedicated trailer for buggies). You don't have to walk through the shop to leave the zoo, so are saved the nightmare 'Can I just have...'

A new 'Children's Village' and play area has just opened (late 2007), and contains a reptile encounter barn, a Golden Lion Tamarin walk-through, and a black rabbit exhibit.'
Maggie, mum of Alice and Katy

Wildfowl and Wetlands Trust Arundel Wetland Centre
Mill Road
Arundel
BN18 9PB
(01903) 883355
info.arundel@wwt.org.uk
www.wwt.org.uk/centre/116/arundel.html

'Great place if you like ducks and geese; we have never seen so many varieties or so many in one place. The Trust is located in a very picturesque setting, along past Arundel Castle. My toddler loved it; you can purchase seed to feed the ducks and geese, which freely wander along the paths. We also took him on the Wetlands boat safari, which he loved. There is a viewing area in the visitors' centre, this has a few toys to offer further distraction; particularly great if the weather is bad. A gift shop, restaurant and toilets are also located in the visitors' centre.'
Jo, mum of Oliver and Jake

Places to Visit

ZSL Whipsnade Zoo
Dunstable
Bedfordshire
LU6 2LF
(01582) 872171
www.zsl.org

'This is about an hour's drive from Guildford. The zoo is quite large, so there is quite a bit of walking to see all the animals, but it is possible to take your car in and drive around the zoo. There is also a little steam train, which goes around the site, and is a good way of seeing some of the animals. There is a small farm and a good playground.

It is quite an expensive day out, but good fun. We found a *Harvester* restaurant between the M1 and the zoo, which is a useful place to stop for dinner on the way home.'
Louise, mum of Joseph and Emilia

Garden Centres

Badshot Lea Garden Centre
Badshot Lea Road
Farnham
GU9 9JX
(01252) 333666
info@badshotlea.net
www.badshotlea.net

'Great for a rainy day as there is a large aquarium containing a variety of coloured fish with many of the tanks at buggy height. There is also a pet centre with guinea pigs, rabbits and mice.

The garden centre is excellent, offering a range of garden plants. There is a large café and there are also baby-changing facilities.'
Jo, mum of Oliver and Jake

'This extensive garden centre is a lovely place to take children. There is a great pet section to explore, with animals including a selection of reptiles and tropical fish in addition to the usual hamsters, mice, guinea pigs and rabbits. There is a large café with plenty of high chairs, which provides hot and cold drinks and various snacks.'
Liz, mum of Elinor

Clandon Park Garden Centre
West Clandon
GU4 7RQ
(01483) 222925
clandonparkGC@aol.com
www.clandonparkgardencentre.co.uk

'The garden centre is situated along a single-track road (with passing spaces), or via a very pleasant walk from the car park of *Clandon House*. It is a small, friendly place with a separate animal centre that houses reptiles and small pet kennels where you can see various varieties of fluffy creatures including goats.

The staff are friendly, and in the main garden centre the owner's dog often comes around for a stroke. There is also an excellent coffee shop with high chairs and homemade, reasonably-priced cakes, and for children, a few books to look at.'
Heather, mum of Tom

Places to Visit

Notcutts Garden and Pet Centre
Guildford Road
Cranleigh
GU6 8LT
(01483) 274222
cranleigh@notcutts.co.uk
www.notcutts.co.uk

'This is an ideal place to visit when it is raining. There is a large pet centre, perfect for wandering around, with small animals, a large fishpond, and parrots tame enough to stay on their tree in the middle of the centre! And Ella loves looking at all the different coloured fish. In the coffee shop there are a couple of play tables, and at Christmas there is a large section just for Christmas decorations that little people love!'
Lynn, mum of Ella

Pottersline Nursery
Potters Lane
Send
GU23 7JJ
(01483) 222211
enquiries@oaklinegroup.com

'Pottersline is a friendly, new nursery with a vast array of unique Italian specimen plants. There is a children's farm and a coffee shop. You can also buy eggs from the lovely clean chickens on the farm. To get there, take Potters Lane, which is signposted directly off the A3 Northbound from Guildford, and Pottersline is clearly marked, at the junction of Potters Lane and Send Hill.'
Beth, mum of Abigail

'I discovered a small farm yesterday, which is free! (You can donate to help the upkeep of animals if you wish). It is really close to Guildford. If you are lost for something to keep the little one amused for half an hour then it's worth a look. There are many nice potted plants on sale, but it is also a working farm. Drive through to the end for parking, which is really nicely laid out with clean wood chips on the floor. There are rabbits, ducks, goats, turkeys, chickens, pigs, Highland cattle and coming soon – wallabies! There is a trampoline set into the ground, which is wicked fun! There is also a coffee shop.'
Jo, mum of Ruby

Secretts Garden Centre
Chapel Lane
Milford
Godalming
GU8 5HU
(01483) 520500
www.secretts.co.uk
[Secretts, at its garden centre site, also has a small wooden play area for children.]

'*Secretts Garden Centre* is a lovely place to visit for an afternoon. You can have a potter around the wide range of plants, both in and outdoors, and feed the ducks on the pond. During the summer, there are usually rabbits playing in a pen by the pond. There is a large café, serving a wide range of drinks, lovely cakes, sandwiches and hot meals. There are plenty of high chairs and usually lots of families around on weekends. On the opposite side of the

Places to Visit

site [by the farm shop] there is a more traditional tearoom selling beautiful gifts and cards, which has high chairs, but is a little less family-oriented. There is also a well-stocked farm shop and 'pick-your-own' fruit and vegetables in the summer months.'
Liz, mum of Elinor

'Both sites (garden centre and farm shop) have a good duck pond to visit and space to toddle around. The garden centre has the more child-friendly café, with sandwiches, fruit and snacks available to buy for toddlers, and plenty of high chairs. That's in addition to the great range of food, plants and gifts available for purchase!'
Heather, mum of Jessica

Squires Garden Centre
Epsom Road
West Horsley
KT24 6AR
(01483) 282911
www.squiresgardencentres.co.uk

'Not a marathon for adults but for toddlers it's perfect, particularly on a wet day. Park your car and you have two places to visit: garden centre and aquarium [the pet centre has recently closed]. The aquarium has a huge range of fish in tanks, these go right down to the ground so it's very accessible for your toddler. The staff don't seem to mind the steady stream of youngsters but there are signs around reminding everyone not to tap the glass. Then you can head off to the garden centre which has traditional garden centre stuff plus a nice café (there were even a few pots of baby food).'
Sonya, mum of Eleanor and Charles

'Squires is a great rainy-day place. It has a lovely fish centre, with tropical fish, waterfalls, and even talking birds. The garden centre also has plenty to look at and has a good coffee shop with high chairs and great toys. At Christmas it's definitely worth a visit to see the lights and Christmas grotto (free visit to Santa in 2006).'
Heather, mum of Tom

'Great conservatory styled restaurant/café. Does baby jars, has a small toy collection, which has just been updated, lovely gift shop, ample parking and next door to fish shop so lots of real life creatures to ogle. Baby-changing facilities at the rear of the store adjacent to café.'
Vicki, mum of George and Finlay

Wyevale Garden Centre
Egley Road
Mayford
Woking
GU22 0NH
(01483) 714861
www.wyevale.co.uk

'A good garden centre, with a small aquatic area, containing a variety of coloured fish, with many of the tanks at buggy height. As the aquatic area is covered, it is an option for a rainy day. The centre has a café and baby-changing

facilities and a good gift shop with a children's book section.'
Jo, mum of Oliver and Jake

Duck Feeding and Paddling

Abinger Hammer
A25 Guildford – Dorking

'On a hot summer's day, the banks of the stream running through Abinger Hammer (on the A25) are the perfect place to be. Park the car in the little car park off the road by the green [Felday Road], and sit in the shade of the big trees on the bank of the stream, or just lie on the grass and bask in the sun. Take wellies or jellies and go paddling and fishing in the stream. There is a large expanse of grass to run around on and a small play park at the far end (great for older children but nothing for young children). Close to the stream there is a tea shop and a village store that sells ice creams, and if you fancy a stroll you can go and watch the village clock strike the hour. Best on weekdays, it can get very busy at the weekend.'
Jo, mum of Thomas, George and Rebecca

Godalming

'You could easily spend the day at the canal in Godalming. Running alongside the canal, there is a wide, generally well-maintained flat footpath, suitable for double buggies, scooters and even bicycles (if you don't mind your child cycling that close to the canal). The path runs from the back of the library to St Peter & St Paul's Church and the Jack Phillips memorial – both of which are also lovely to look around. There are ducks, swans and geese all the way along the canal, but particularly near the library. The wildlife can get a bit greedy, so sometimes you need to watch out for the rather demanding geese. You can also take the 'footbridge' through the swamp area where you can occasionally see more ducks and maybe a few frogs. At the church end is a big field, which is great for picnics, particularly under the tree, and just behind the bowling green is a lovely playground.'
Emma, mum of Charlotte and Louis

'With easy parking in the large pay and display car park, Godalming is great for an afternoon visit. Only a short walk from the car park there is a lovely park with equipment for all ages. Just beyond this is the river, with a tarmac path winding along beside, where you can feed the ducks. On a cold afternoon it is not too far to stroll into town and grab a coffee in one of the cafés.'
Liz, mum of Elinor

Millmead

'This is a great place to feed the ducks (and the occasional persistent bird). We often walk over the footbridge by *Debenhams* and walk along the canal path watching the barges and wildlife. There is a lovely statue of *Alice in Wonderland*, which my girls have always loved sitting on and play-acting around. You can feed the ducks all along the path and also

Places to Visit

over the other side of the canal. In the summer there is often an ice cream seller parked up and if you are brave you can have a picnic on the benches overlooking the water. Great fun all year round and a nice place to take visitors for a quick stroll.'
Rebecca, mum of Isabelle, Aimee and Robyn

'Most of Surrey's wild fowl hang out behind the Yvonne Arnaud Theatre in Guildford. You can park in Millmead car park and access this area by walking to the left of the theatre and across the bridge. Make sure you take as much bread as possible as it has to go a long way! After feeding the ducks here, why not watch the colourful barges going through the lock or go for a walk towards St Catherine's, along the canal?'
Debra, mum of Ben and Eddie

Pirbright

'There is a car park beside Lord Pirbright Village Hall, next to the playground, which has some good old fashioned swings, slides and roundabouts. From here it is a two-minute walk to the pond, which has an island in the middle, and this year ducks with no less than 10 ducklings. There are benches to sit on and throw bread to them. There is also a resident goose this year (2007) who always seems to be standing in the same place keeping an eye on things, but it hasn't been aggressive.'
Maggie, mum of Alice and Katy

Shere

[Note: there is a playground in Shere behind the Village Hall on Gomshall Lane – see Playgrounds later in this chapter.]

'A picturesque Surrey Hills village only a few miles outside Guildford on the A25. The river is shallow and very clean and ducks are plentiful. Many children paddle in the water in the heat of summer. There is also a lovely, flat and easy-to-navigate walk that takes you along the river towards the Albury Estate. Shere's toilets, public houses and shops are all nearby.'
Debra, mum of Ben and Eddie

'One very, very hot summer day we drove to Shere and spent a good half hour just wading in the river where it flows through town. It was cool and shady, there were ducks paddling about, and one of the shops in Shere sells ice creams. Amazing how just putting your feet in cool water changes your mood and energies completely!'
Kris, mum of Olivia and Victoria

'If you're lucky with parking, it's a great way to spend some time. You can play 'Poohsticks' on a tiny bridge over the ford. It depends how busy the village has been that day as to how hungry ducks are, but you can buy bags of bread at the nearby café, the *Lucky Duck*, if you've forgotten to bring some (it's also a nice place to eat). The stream is also shallow enough to wade about in wellies.'
Sonya, mum of Eleanor and Charles

Surrey University
GU2 7XH

'If you walk to the centre of the University of Surrey campus, there's a large pleasant lake with lots of big carp and ducks to feed. There are also many grassy areas nearby for running around or playing ball. We then usually go up the hill to the cathedral and have a drink in the refectory.'
Julie, mum of Ben and Katie

National Trust (NT) Houses and Gardens
[Please note that you can find information on all NT venues on the same website: www.nationaltrust.org.uk]

'I would thoroughly recommend joining the *National Trust* – we are extremely lucky in this area to have so many NT properties close to hand and the membership soon pays for itself after a few visits. At £72.50 for 2007 joint annual membership (for two adults, under-fives go free), with just over five visits your membership will have paid for itself. They are great places to meet friends or else to just pop out for a quick walk. All have excellent facilities for babies – changing, food warming etc.'
Karen, mum of Ewan

'Good value if you become a member as you can pop in for an hour without resenting a high entry charge. There is always something on during the school and bank holidays. Properties are mostly closed in winter, which is a pity.'
Sonya, mum of Eleanor and Charles

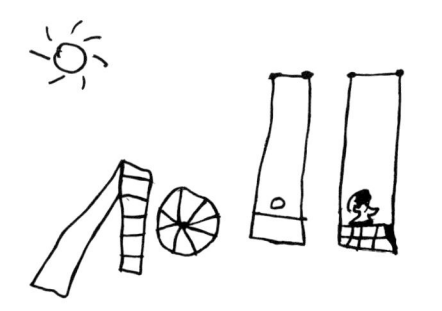

Clandon Park
West Clandon
GU4 7RQ
(01483) 222482
clandonpark@nationaltrust.org.uk

'This *National Trust* property is a beautifully quiet place just outside of Guildford. The gardens are small but have plenty of places for a toddler to run about and explore safely. There are paths suitable for pushchairs around the property but if entering the house you have to leave your buggy at the entrance; there is a supply of baby-carriers available for use, however. The house is interesting for both adults and older children, with a quiz available to maintain older children's interest. There are baby-changing facilities, a restaurant on site, or you can wander up to the garden centre to use its café. Check opening times, as it is seasonal. It is closed

Places to Visit

on a lot of Saturdays and some Fridays for weddings.'
Heather, mum of Tom

'Clandon Park is a lovely place for a walk and the café in the garden centre is an ideal place for a cup of tea and a slice of homemade cake! The pet centre, which is situated near to the garden centre, has goats outside which the kids, excuse the pun, will love.'
Karen, mum of Ewan

'Visit *Clandon Park* for its quizzes and trails, some of which are year-round and some seasonal or for special events.'
Sonya, mum of Eleanor and Charles

'Lovely to spend a morning or afternoon here. Park up and have a walk around the grounds and then pop along to the garden centre where there is a very friendly café. Also great for kids is the fish aquarium, which will keep them captivated for ages.'
Avril, mum of Scarlett

Claremont Landscape Gardens
Portsmouth Road
Esher
KT10 9JG
(01372) 467806
claremont@nationaltrust.org.uk

'This is a lovely place to go for a walk. It is a nice size, enough room to run around in, but you can walk around most of the park without smaller legs getting too exhausted. The paths are buggy-friendly and the bulk of the park around the lake is fairly flat; however, the steeper side is still quite easy to navigate with a buggy. There is a large lake with geese and ducks, which you can feed, and there is a children's play area.'
Katherine, mum of Holly and Hazel

'Lovely place to walk with a pushchair or with toddlers. It has a large pool that you can circle while feeding the birds (ducks, geese and swans) with hidden seats that you discover around each corner. Has different activities during the holiday season – we attended a teddy bear picnic and art activities last year. Nice sheltered coffee shop (where babies were cooed over) and you can dine both inside or alfresco.'
Vicki, mum of George and Finlay

Dapdune Wharf
Wharf Road
GU1 4RR
(01483) 561389
riverwey@nationaltrust.org.uk
[Dapdune Wharf is part of almost 20 miles of River Wey and Godalming Navigations.]

'A great little museum with plenty of interactive exhibits. There is also a boat trip from *Dapdune Wharf* to Millmead, which is a lovely way to see the river and an interesting way to approach the town centre. The coffee shop is basic, but there's a nice picnic area. The waterway runs right next to the museum, so you need to watch the kids extra carefully.'
Julie, mum of Ben and Katie

Places to Visit

Hatchlands Park
East Clandon
GU4 7RT
(01483) 222482
hatchlands@nationaltrust.org.uk

'We have visited *Hatchlands* since Tom was a baby. We have not yet made it into the house as we tend to go for walks through the extensive parkland instead. There are many benches dotted about for toddler rests and various lengths of walks to suit all. I would particularly recommend visiting at bluebell time as the bluebell wood is spectacular. I have managed to do all the walks with my pushchair although it does have rough terrain wheels and the paths require it in parts. There is a restaurant and toilets with baby-changing facilities situated by the house.'
Heather, mum of Tom

'*Hatchlands Park* is ideal if you fancy some fresh air - there is an area of the park that is full of bluebells in the spring, which is beautiful. There is plenty of open space and some amazing views out to London. The cows are also free to wander the parkland - so you need to watch your step!'
Karen, mum of Ewan

'Visit *Hatchlands* around March/April time for the fabulous daffodils, and May for the wonderful bluebells. It's definitely worth doing the Easter egg trails/quizzes.'
Sonya, mum of Eleanor and Charles

Mottisfont Abbey
(Garden, House & Estate)
Mottisfont
nr Romsey
Hampshire
SO51 0LP
(01794) 340757
motissfontabbey@nationaltrust.org.uk

'This *National Trust* property is about an hour and a quarter's drive from Guildford, but if you choose a day when there is a special children's activity or family event, it's well worth the journey. There is usually an artist in residence who often runs some really great workshops. Look on the NT website for details of events. We always go there in late September to make the most of the conker harvest. The kids come away with carrier bags that are so full they can barely lift them! Other highlights include rolling races down the grassy banks, walks along the river where you can watch the large fish in crystal-clear water, and playing hide and seek around the walled rose garden. The house is worth a visit too, and it has a good tearoom.'
Jo, mum of Thomas, George and Rebecca

Polesden Lacey
Great Bookham
RH5 6BD
(01372) 452048
polesdenlacey@nationaltrust.org.uk

'*Polesden Lacey* has always been a favourite of our family's. There is something about the enormous expanse of green lawn

Places to Visit

sloping down from the house that cries out to the child in all of us; in the summer months, this lawn is fairly littered with picnickers, families, gatherings of all kinds, and people of all ages enjoying the atmosphere. There are walks of varying lengths and descriptions, breathtaking views, astounding flower gardens, and a wonderful tearoom, with a courtyard fountain, which you will be hard pressed to keep your children from throwing themselves into. *Polesden Lacey* also plays host to a wide variety of seasonal events: country fairs, evening entertainments, children's activities, Christmas craft fairs, themed weekends (apple harvest, chocolate) and the like. The tearoom does children's meals.'
Kris, mum of Olivia and Victoria

'This is situated close to Dorking and comprises a beautiful house and lots of gardens. Pushchairs are not allowed in the house, however the gardens are open to everyone and there of lots of different walks available (most suitable for pushchairs). My family loves going here in the spring/summer with a picnic.'
Becki, mum of Jack

'*Polesden Lacey* is stunning and there are trails for children as well as family-activity packs. On a sunny day it is the perfect place to take a picnic and sit on the expanse of lawn in front of the house and either relax and enjoy the beautiful vistas of the North Downs or else join in with the 'roly polies' down the hill.'
Karen, mum of Ewan

Winkworth Arboretum
Hascombe Road
Godalming
GU8 4AD
(01483) 208477
winkwortharbortetum@nationaltrust.org.uk

'*Winkworth* is a *National Trust* arboretum just near Godalming. It's a lovely place for a walk, and is particularly stunning when the bluebells are out, and in the autumn when the trees are gorgeous colours. Parts of it are quite steep and hilly but the map shows paths that avoid steps, and there are walks you can do that are fairly flat and easy with a buggy. There are lakes and a boat-house, and the café does great cream teas. We've never used the baby-changing facilities, but according to the website they are there!'
Jo, mum of James and Daisy

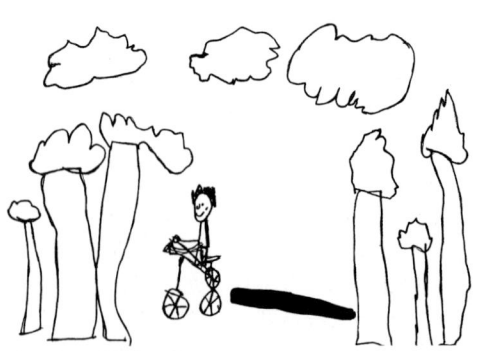

'This is located about two miles from Godalming and is part of the *National Trust*. It is great to go to at all times of year as the scenery is ever-changing. My son Jack loves it. There are lots of different walks available and also lots of open areas for picnics.'
Becki, mum of Jack

Parks and Gardens

Bushey Park
Hampton Court Road
TW12 2EJ
(020) 8979 1586
bushy@royalparks.gsi.gov.uk
www.royalparks.gov.uk/parks/bushy_park

'One of our favourite trips is to *Bushey Park*. It has pretty much everything you could hope for in a London park. Lots of ponds and streams with swans and ducks for the little ones to feed, a fantastic playground with big slides, a huge sandpit (bring your own bucket and spade, or *Scoop* and *Muck*!), a free car park, a hut that sells rather excellent hot drinks, ice cream and sandwiches, lots of nooks and crannies to explore, and deer. We like to run-off steam in the playground and then cross the road over to *Hampton Court* to wander around the free gardens there or walk by the river. The *Hampton Court* gardens are gorgeous in spring-time when they are covered in daffodils. The café at *Hampton Court* has lots of space, a baby-changing area and good seating outside, but is a little pricey.'
Jacqui, mum of Harry and Megan

Denbies Wine Estate
London Road
Dorking
RH5 6AA
(01306) 876616
www.denbiesvineyard.co.uk

'*Denbies* is a local favourite for mums and babes and retirees too. Outdoors is fantastic for long strolls with the pushchair. The 'train path' leads you for hours of walks around the vines. Overall, it is child-friendly and great for Sunday afternoon family entertainment. Indoors, there is a very spacious casual eating area under a huge atrium. We always have to sit at a table next to the fishpond for my son. There is a good variety of cold and warm food and plenty of cakes! The gift shop is great around Christmas or Easter for those special decorations or gifts. Do the tour with wine tastings for adults and train ride (indoors and outdoors) for children.'
Fabienne, mum of Louis and Margaux

Guildford Castle Grounds
Castle Street
GU1 3TU
(01483) 444718
museum@guildford.gov.uk
www.guildford.gov.uk/Guildfordweb/Tourism

'The castle grounds are particularly lovely in the summer, when the well-manicured landscaped gardens are in full bloom. Charlotte and Louis love running around, smelling the flowers, exploring the narrow pathways and staircases, and of course gazing at the castle. We often enter a land of fantasy, telling stories of the princes and princesses who live in the castle. In addition, the views from the castle are lovely. If you're lucky you may be serenaded by a small orchestra practising in the bandstand near to the bowling green.

It's also good fun to spend an evening with friends watching the Shakespeare plays that are performed by *Guildford Shakespeare Company* over a few weeks every summer.'
Emma, mum of Charlotte and Louis

'Always a lovely colourful place to either push babies around, let them crawl or when they are older run around.'
Leena, mum of Ella

Hampton Court Palace
KT8 9AU
(0870) 752 7777
hamptoncourt@hrp.org.uk
www.hrp.org.uk

'This was surprisingly easy to get to on a Sunday morning. Parking in the grounds costs £3.00 [in 2007], and that allows you to walk through the gardens and then out on to the Thames towpath. In the gardens, there is a large restaurant, which is child-friendly, has a large selection of food, high chairs and a clean baby-changing room. We didn't venture into the Palace but walking and eating was a perfect day out in itself!'
Lynn and Paul, parents of Ella

Kew Gardens
Royal Botanic Gardens
Kew
Richmond
TW9 3AB
(020) 8332 5655
info@kew.org
www.kew.org

'Trips to *Kew Gardens* have been winners every time for us. We particularly enjoy climbing, sliding and digging in 'Climbers and Creepers' [an interactive botanical play zone], crawling in and out of the badger sett, watching fish in the aquarium and riding the 'Kew Explorer'. The cafés are great too!'
Hilary, mum of Oliver and Ben

Loseley Park
GU3 1HS
(01483) 304440
www.loseley-park.com

'A great place to visit during the summer months, where you can wander round the beautiful walled gardens or simply sit in the grounds and sample the fantastic *Loseley* ice cream or enjoy a picnic. To the far right of the walled garden is an open waterway, so young children will need supervision, but the waterway is very picturesque and you can usually spot some wildlife (moorhens) on there to keep them amused. There is a small adventure playground next to the car park and a lake to walk down to, although this not particularly buggy-friendly. There is a small café and baby-changing facilities. During September, *Loseley* has the added

advantage of being free for *RHS Wisley* cardholders.'
Jo, mum of Oliver and Jake

Painshill Park
Portsmouth Road
Cobham
KT11 1JE
(01932) 868113
info@painshill.co.uk
www.painshill.co.uk

'The entrance is nestled between houses on a main road in Cobham. However, this inconspicuous entrance opens out into a fantastic space and parkland beyond. The grounds are well-maintained with a lake, vines, a grotto, bridges and a ruin; and there is a map for children to use to navigate around the lake. There is also a good selection of birds on the lakes that my children like watching. Watch out for seasonal activities at *Painshill Park* such as Father Christmas and Easter Parades etc. It makes a good day out.'
Debra, mum of Ben and Eddie

Ramster
Chiddingfold,
GU8 4SN
(01428) 654167 (office hours only)
www.ramsterevents.com

'Historical manor house with gardens to walk in, and a very family-friendly tea shop [open April – June 10.00 am – 5.00 pm daily] with toys and space for children to run around.'
Paige, mum of Miranda and Leo

Richmond Park
TW10 5HS
(020) 8948 3209
richmond@royalparks.gsi.gov.uk
www.royalparks.gov.uk/parks/richmond_park/

'The open spaces, woods, ponds, deer and parakeets make *Richmond Park* a wonderful place for families to explore. We love walking and kite-flying there, and also cycling as there is a great variety of designated cycle paths. Bikes with all the children's accessories can be hired within the park.'
Hilary, mum of Oliver and Ben

Windsor Great Park
Windsor
SL4 2HT
(01753) 860222
enquiries@thecrownestate.co.uk
www.thecrownestate.co.uk/1651_the_windsor_great_park

'A great location for a picnic and for simply enjoying the outdoors. You can access the park via Virginia Water, which itself offers lovely walks and is great pram-pushing country! We often choose to park in the *Savill Gardens* car park and access the park via the path situated to the left of the car park entrance. From here you can easily walk though the *Great Park* down to Virginia Water. *Windsor Great Park* is popular so it can get busy in the summer.

There are restaurant and baby-changing facilities located in *Savill Gardens*, which

in turn is also worth a visit, although entrance to these gardens is not free.'
Jo, mum of Oliver and Jake

Wisley RHS Garden
Woking
GU23 6QB
(0845) 260 9000
info@rhs.org.uk
www.rhs.org.uk/gardens/wisley

'Audrey loves getting out of her pushchair to walk along the paths of this beautiful garden. Her favourite game is chasing after the ducks. There is a child-friendly cafeteria near the entrance with several high chairs (though sometimes not quite enough for the many children there), changing facilities, and a play area (in a marquee attached to the building, so it can be quite cold, loud and not always very clean in there). All in all though, a lovely morning out, and let's not forget the wonderful shop on the way out!'
Kelley, mum of Audrey

'This is an easy place to walk with a buggy, and we visited so often I became a member (this entitles you plus one guest to enter, and children under six are free). There are several walks, and clearly signposted paths for buggies and wheelchairs. There are two cafés: one in the woods, and the main restaurant, which has a selection of hot and cold food, and tempting cakes and drinks. There is also a microwave to heat baby food. Lunchtime can get very busy, but there is usually a good supply of high chairs. There is a small play area in the (non-heated) marquee for toddlers to have a run-around. There are a few baby-change toilets both around the gardens and within the restaurant complex. A great way to appreciate the changing seasons with frequent visits. You have to get there early to get a parent and child parking space!'
Heather, mum of Jessica

'RHS membership entitles the member to unlimited access with one adult guest or two children six to 16 years and little ones (under six) are free. We go there regularly as there is plenty of space for children to run around (and no worry about dog mess, unlike some of the woodland dog walking areas!) Lots to look at, with a huge variety of flowers, trees and plants, and some fountains/ponds with a few ducks and fish. There are plenty of flat paths and ramps so the access is excellent for buggies. The café has a nice selection of food, although is a little on the expensive side.'
Lisa, mum of Thomas

Walks and Family Cycling

Alice Holt Forest
Bucks Horn Oak
Nr Farnham
GU10 4LS
(01420) 520212 (recreation officer)
kathleen.calver@forestry.gsi.gov.uk
www.forestry.gov.uk/aliceholt

'*Alice Holt* has been a hit with everyone I've taken there. Forest tracks make

Places to Visit

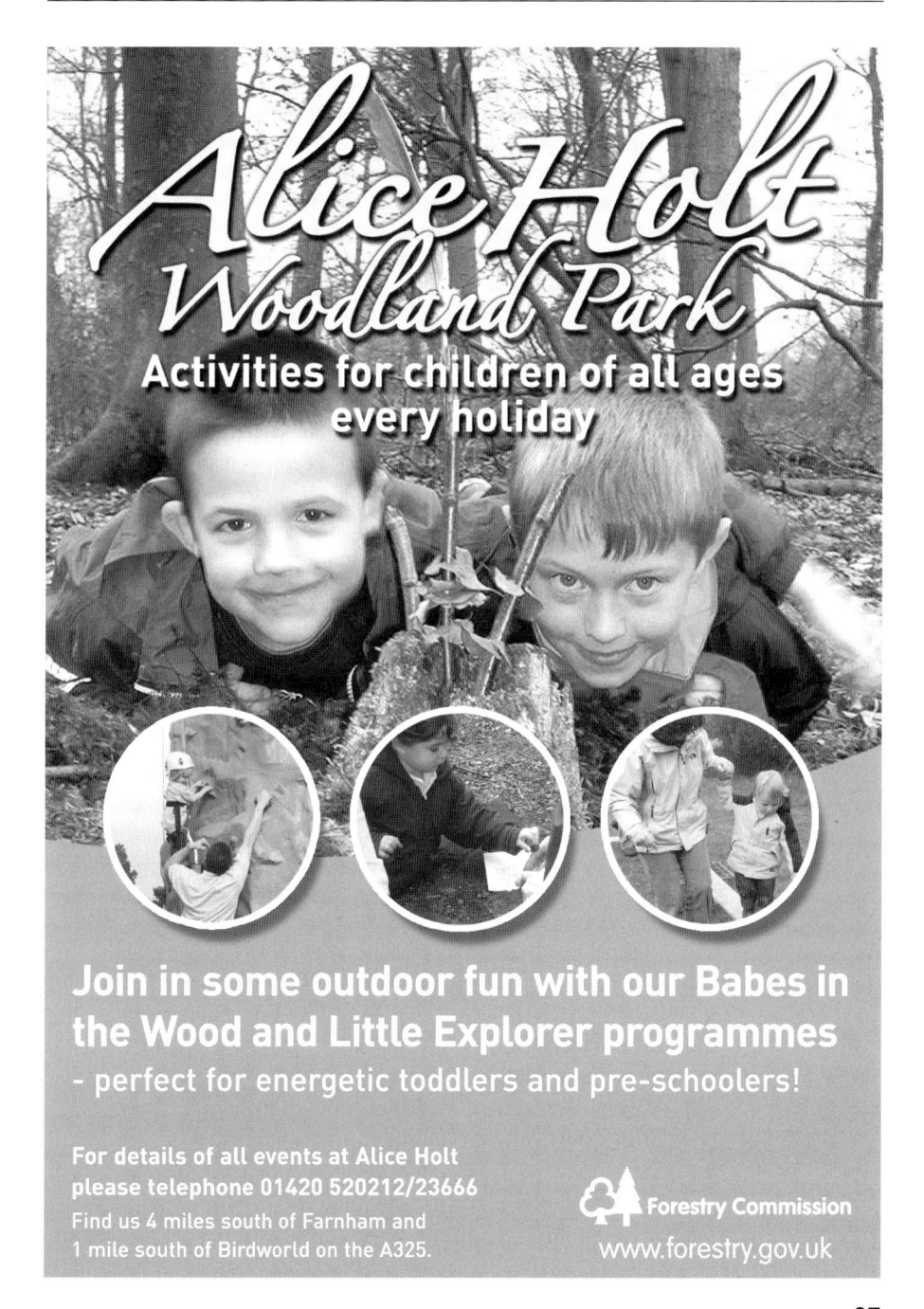

Alice Holt Woodland Park

Activities for children of all ages every holiday

Join in some outdoor fun with our Babes in the Wood and Little Explorer programmes
- perfect for energetic toddlers and pre-schoolers!

For details of all events at Alice Holt
please telephone 01420 520212/23666
Find us 4 miles south of Farnham and
1 mile south of Birdworld on the A325.

Forestry Commission
www.forestry.gov.uk

suitable walks for prams and pushchairs, [off-roaders are best], and there are a few climbing frames along some of the paths to encourage small children to keep going, although it was searching for fungi that kept my niece and nephew's legs moving.

There are also three adventure playgrounds: one with swings for small children next to a large grassy area, another which my seven-year-old nephew was old enough to enjoy most of, and then a new high-wire 'Go Ape' course for very brave over-tens. You can cycle round the forest, hiring bikes and kiddie trailers if you need to. There are many organised activities including climbing, den building, and welly races (check the website for dates and details).

The visitors' centre sells a map showing the facilities, has toilets, baby-change facilities, and sells drinks and snacks.'
Fiona, mum of Thomas

'Fantastic day out in good weather. A variety of marked trails – buy a map from the shop. The shortest one with the adventure playgrounds is best for younger kids. You can take bikes but there are a few hilly bits that adults will need to push young bikers up – brace your backs!

There is a newly refurbished coffee shop selling food too. Car park is £3.00 for the day, pay and display – well worth it. Unless weather has been dry for a while, wear wellies and take change of trousers and shoes for afterwards. Excellent outdoor fun.'
Helen, mum of Dominic and Laura

Chantry Wood
Pilgrims Way
Guildford

'If you park in the car park off Pilgrims Way you can do a simple circular walk. Start by heading up the steep chalky path heading into the woods. Follow this track along the edge of the wood, giving nice views over the fields. At the top, there is a lovely clearing with a tree that is wonderful for climbing and bouncing on. Then you can head back down the hill along a different path (although going in a very similar direction), which brings you back out by the car park. There are paths all over the place so you can make your walk as long or as short as you want. There are some stunning views over the Wey Valley and in bluebell time you can come across some wonderful patches of colour.'
Jo, mum of Thomas, George and Rebecca

Church of St. Martha-on-the-hill
Access via public footpaths, about ¾ mile from car parks on Halfpenny Lane and Guildford Lane

'The Church itself is open weekends and bank holidays, but the churchyard is always open. The walks there from the car parks have truly spectacular views, so are always worth the climb. The church is located at the top of a very steep hill on the Chantries [the summit is about 530 ft], but as the terrain is very steep I do not think it is very practical for pushchairs.'
Becki, mum of Jack

Places to Visit

Compton Woods
Polsted Lane

'If you visit Compton Woods towards the end of April or beginning of May you are sure of a wonderful display of bluebells. You can park right by the woods and although the initial bit of the path can be very muddy, it's usually fine once you get into the woods proper. The woods are quite small so are perfect for a stroll with a toddler. You simply meander around the little paths in the wood or stick to the main track. They are not really suitable for buggies. There is a tiny stream running through the woods, and loads of badger setts for added interest. To get to the woods, drive through Compton from the A3 and turn left into Polsted Lane. Continue along here for a little way and then pull up and park on the verge opposite the allotments where you see a footpath heading into the woodland on your left.'
Jo, mum of Thomas, George and Rebecca

Guildford Cathedral
Stag Hill
GU2 7UP
(01483) 547860
reception@guildford-cathedral.org
www.guildford-cathedral.org

'A nice walk that we like to do on a clear day is up to the cathedral. The hill is a little steep, but great exercise and has good views of Guildford from the top. If it's a little cold or wet outside, a venture inside the cathedral has lots to offer. Check out the occasional lunchtime concerts. There is also a café in the building next to the cathedral, which offers a decent range of food and drinks and has high chairs.'
Jacqui, mum of Harry and Megan

'On Saturday afternoons there are often final rehearsals taking place for that evening's concert so you can take the children along to see a full orchestra in motion. In the case of *Vivace Chorus* concerts, you get 130 singers as well as the orchestra! My two absolutely love it and, unlike at a concert, it doesn't matter if they make a noise as the cathedral is fully open to the public during the rehearsals. Kieron (four) loves going right up to the drums and counting how many sticks they have and sometimes likes to pretend to conduct the choir! Trumpets are a firm favourite with him too, although Anthony (one) isn't too sure of them yet. It's much better than a real concert when you have to sit still!'
Miranda, mum of Kieron and Anthony

Family cycling
(0845) 113 0065
info@sustrans.org.uk
www.sustrans.co.uk

'There are various off-road cycle routes in the area that can all be found on the *Sustrans* website. For ease, we tend to go on the old railway line that now runs from Peasmarsh to Brighton. We usually join it at Bramley because there is a car park right next to the track. Coming from Guildford, you get to it by turning

left at the first roundabout in Bramley then go a short way along the road until you see the car park at the old station on your left. From there you can go in either direction either back towards Guildford or out towards Cranleigh. It's a traffic-free, reasonably flat surface and some nice views. Sometimes we start from Cranleigh, and if you head away from Guildford you reach a pub before too long, which is fine for a drink and a packet of crisps before heading home.'
Jo, mum of Thomas, George and Rebecca

Frensham Pond
Bacon Lane
Churt
Farnham
GU10 2QB
www.waverley.gov.uk/countryside/frenshampond.asp

'This is about 20 minutes from Guildford, and is lovely for walks or a spot of swimming, paddling and sunbathing in the summer. When we first went, we were amazed at the beautiful sandy beach that kept Harry very entertained. You can swim in the ponds; a notice-board next to the pond keeps you informed as to the water quality, which has generally been very good whenever we have gone. If you prefer something a little more exerting, then there are a number of well-signposted trails, and an information centre next to the car park gives you more information about the history of the area and wildlife to look out for. There is a refreshment hut that offers burgers, drinks and ice creams. The car park is free in the winter and during off-peak times.'
Jacqui, mum of Harry and Megan

'We love going here when the weather permits. There is a little beach area by a lake where children (and adults) can play. The setting is lovely and unspoilt. There is a hut selling refreshments, and reasonable toilet facilities. This is a must for those who want a beach without travelling all the way to the coast. It is possible to swim in the water but you must check the warning sign for [blue-green] algae as it changes. There is not much shade so best to bring a parasol.'
Thora, mum of Freyja

Friday Street
Abinger Common
Dorking
RH5 6JR

'From the main *National Trust* car park on Friday Street, walk down the hill until you reach the lake at the bottom. Keep walking with the lake on your right, and at the bottom of the hill there is a gap in the fence on the right, signposted as a footpath. Stay on the lower path close to the water's edge (a nice place for a picnic). This eventually reaches a good clearing in the woods, which is great for making camps. My eldest son (seven) said that he had 'found paradise' and while my idea of paradise is a cocktail, and white sandy beach, I could see his point! My boys played here for ages. After a stop, continue along the path away from the lake and you will get to a bridge over a stream. Turn right here and you return to the hamlet of Friday Street, but there are many other walks that you could take from this point too.

If you want to combine a walk with lunch with the kids then you can try the *Stephan Langton* pub in Friday Street itself. While it does not have a children's menu, there are one or two 'safe' options such as sausage and mash. It does get quite busy so booking is recommended.

For those with older children, rather than taking the lower path, take the one that leads up the hill and through the trees. You will eventually get to a waterfall that the children will enjoy, but I would suggest that this is not for children under the age of seven.'
Debra, mum of Ben and Eddie

Newlands Corner
Shere Road
Guildford
GU4 8SE
www.guildford.gov.uk/GuildfordWeb/Tourism

'This can be the start of a long or short walk, or is a destination in itself to have a snack or ice cream at the refreshment stand. It is right off the A25 towards Shere. There are toilets, baby-changing facilities and plenty of free parking with picnic tables, and lots of lovely grass for spreading out a picnic blanket and enjoying the stunning views of downs and woodland.'
Kelley, mum of Audrey

Sheepleas
Shere Road
West Horsley

'The routes through Sheepleas take in grassy fields, woods and meadows, yet in fine weather can easily be traversed by a buggy (might not be so easy following wet weather). There's plenty of space for running about, great dens that have been built in the woods, tree climbing and a big picnic area with tables. It's a great place for a walk and for burning off some energy.

Take the A246, Epsom Road out of Guildford towards Leatherhead. At the Bell & Coleville Garage roundabout, turn right, sign posted Sheepleas and go along for about half a mile, before you come to a car park on the left-hand side.'
Julie, mum of Ben and Katie

Whitmoor Common
Salt Box Road
Worplesdon

'This common is situated between Guildford and Woking, and is best accessed via Salt Box Road. It is enclosed roughly by Salt Box Road to the South, Worplesdon Road to the West, Burdenshott Road to the East, and Goose Rye Road to the North, with the main railway line running through it. It is a Specially Protected Area and a Site of Specific Scientific Interest, and one of the common's main features is its large expanse of heathland that is home to large quantities of flora and fauna. It is a flat, sandy common that is very prone to flooding, so wear appropriate footwear depending on the weather. There are numerous paths criss-crossing the common, so it's easy to pick a route appropriate to your needs. If you're feeling energetic, you can walk to *The Jolly Farmer* on Burdenshott Rd which is ideal for young families in the summer with its huge beer garden.

One of the Common's main attractions from my son Ben's point of view is the footbridge over the railway line, which provides a great vantage point for train-watching – the drivers usually oblige by tooting the horn. Extremely popular with dog-walkers, so you can always guarantee meeting lots of four-legged friends. What it lacks in dramatic scenery, it makes up for with convenience and accessibility.'
Bill, dad of Ben and Ella

Trips and Days Out
Museums and Exhibitions

Amberley Working Museum
West Sussex
BN18 9LT
(01798) 831370
www.amberleymuseum.co.uk

'This is a strange museum built in an old chalk pit. It appears to be much-loved by our grandparents' generation who love reminiscing over things from their childhood. However, it also has a great deal to interest the children. For starters it has 'free' (donations expected) rides on vintage vehicles and a narrow-gauge railway. There are several trails for children and one or two days each week, during school holidays, the education room is open. On the day we went, this was full of interesting activities including printing, drawing, handling artefacts, making models to demonstrate how chalk was formed, and quizzes. You could also borrow art equipment and enter the art competition, make something with clay at the potter's, print a poster at the printer's, watch various craftsmen in action and have plenty of refreshments in the newly built café area.

At just over an hour's drive from Guildford (through beautiful countryside) this is well worth a visit, but look at the website and make sure you go on a day when the education room is open – and don't forget to take the grandparents, they'll love it!'
Jo, mum of Thomas, George and Rebecca

Beaulieu Abbey and Motor Museum
John Montagu Building
Brockenhurst
Hampshire
SO42 7ZN
(01590) 612345
www.beaulieu.co.uk

'We discovered this place one summer while camping at Round Hill campsite in the New Forest, (which, by the way, in my opinion is the best family campsite in the New Forest even though is doesn't have showers); but the journey is very do-able in a day trip from Guildford. Although it was expensive, we got our money's worth because you can convert your one-day ticket into a two-day pass at no extra cost as long as your second visit is within the week. Even after two days, we were still discovering more things to do.

We loved the monorail, which takes you through the roof of the motor museum and over the Victorian garden where the kids tried in vain to get the Victorian gardener to wave to them. We also enjoyed the ride-through exhibit in the motor museum and choosing our favourite cars from the hundreds on display. We loved seeing the vintage cars driving around and seeing the man mount his penny-farthing bicycle was a real education! We would have got more out of the *PlayStation* Dome if we'd known what we were doing, but the display about training the secret agents during WWII was fascinating.

What I loved was the huge range of things on offer. From learning about the history of the Abbey and watching Victorian re-enactments in the house, to relaxing in the garden and being a car geek, there really is something for everyone.'
Jo, mum of Thomas, George and Rebecca

Brooklands Museum
Brooklands Road
Weybridge
KT13 0QN
(01932) 857381
info@brooklandsmuseum.com
www.brooklandsmuseum.com
[See also review for *Mercedes-Benz World* later in this chapter.]

'Accessed via the recently opened Mercedes-Benz World, the *Brooklands Museum* is a good distraction for an afternoon or morning's activity. Indoor exhibits include racing cars, bikes and automobiles. Outside exhibits include *Concorde*, passenger planes and buses, all of which you can view from the inside.

Good for a showery day too as a fair proportion of the museum is inside. In the summer, racing cars are often on display and offer adult passenger trips round the infamous racing circuit. A restaurant and baby-changing facilities are available at the museum.'
Jo, mum of Oliver and Jake

Guildford House Gallery
155 High Street
GU1 3AJ
(01483) 444740/2
guildfordhouse@guildford.gov.uk
www.guildford.gov.uk/guildfordweb/ leisure/guildfordhouse

'*Guildford House Gallery* is always worth a quick visit if you're passing. Entry is free and the exhibitions change every few months, some being of more interest to children than others. There is always a well-equipped art trolley to amuse the children and on the upstairs landing, there are some lovely cushions to sit on and a box of children's books. Downstairs there is a small tearoom, and the shop is full of beautiful things but not somewhere you can let a toddler roam! Look out for the art workshops that the gallery sometimes runs for older children and the occasional family art day (e.g. The Big Draw).'
Jo, mum of Thomas, George and Rebecca

Places to Visit

Haslemere Museum
78 High Street
Haslemere
GU27 2LA
(01428) 642112
enquiries@haslemeremuseum.co.uk
www.haslemeremuseum.co.uk

'Haslemere Museum is a great little museum, really geared up for kids. It contains a huge assortment of exhibits from fossils and natural history to an Egyptian mummy and Victorian clothes (some can be tried on!) Outside there is a 'living hive' exhibit where you can look inside a beehive and watch the bees at work. There is also a short walk around the grounds that takes in a pond and various follies. The museum doesn't take very long to go around but it has children's trails and activity bags that children can borrow and take around with them. It also has a small but well-stocked shop. It is housed in a lovely old building in the High Street, so it's easy to park nearby and walk to.'
Jo, mum of Thomas, George and Rebecca

INTECH Science and Discovery Centre
Telegraph Way
Morn Hill
Winchester
SO21 1HX
(01962) 863791
htct@intech-uk.com
www.intech-uk.com

'At 40 minutes straight down the A31 INTECH is very easy to get to. It's probably aimed at the five to 12 age range, but if younger children are 'in tow' there's plenty there to keep them amused. Every exhibit is a hands-on demonstration of a scientific principle, very similar to the Launch Pad area in the Science Museum in London, but INTECH is bigger. You can purchase several very interesting trails to help older children be focused during their visit. There is also a lecture theatre/planetarium that has science shows several times a day. When we went, there was a very interesting show all about optical illusions. There is also a restaurant and a picnic area. Entrance isn't cheap but if you're looking for a trip to interest older children while at the same time amusing younger children this is a good place to go.'
Jo, mum of Thomas, George and Rebecca

The Look Out Discovery Centre
Nine Mile Ride
Bracknell
RG12 7QW
(01344) 354400
thelookout@bracknell-forest.gov.uk
www.bracknell-forest.gov.uk/lookout

'My kids and I love the *Look Out Centre*. It is a science discovery centre for children, primarily targeted, I think, at school-age children. However, my two and four-year-olds love playing with the boats, operating the locks, working out the food chain, running up and down the giant piano, releasing the hot air balloon, putting together the body, making badges…I could go on. Outdoors there is a lovely wooden playground, and you can hire

bikes to browse the acres of woodland within which the centre is set. Oh, and I mustn't forget the Look Out tower, which I must confess I haven't yet brought myself round to climbing with two such little ones. But I will; the views must be lovely. The café is extremely reasonably-priced with unique pop-up animals (near the ceiling in the conservatory) to keep the kids entertained while they are eating!'
Emma, mum of Charlotte and Louis

'This is a great family day out. The *Discovery Centre* is set in the middle of a wood (which Daddies love to go cycling in!) and has a great outside rustic playground. Inside the centre there are loads of things for children of all ages to do. It is a bit like a mini Science Museum with hands on areas looking at water, nature, light, sound and much more. My boys who are two and four (and thirty-five!) love it. For lunch you can either take a picnic (there are loads of picnic tables) or there is a small café there. There is also a cycle hire centre for the more adventurous.'
Sarah, mum of Zack and Fin

RAF Museum London
Grahame Park Way
Hendon
NW9 5LL
(020) 8205 2266
london@rafmuseum.org
www.rafmuseum.org.uk

'Definitely one for the boys! My two sons, now five and seven, have frequently visited this museum and never seem to tire of it. It is a bit of a walk from the tube station, so I would suggest driving and there is a good-sized car park. The range of aircraft on display is fantastic and the kids love the interactive play area. Some of the exhibits can be clambered on, which make this even more exciting for the children. There is a small café area on-site for basic food requirements, however a picnic area is also provided.'
Debra, mum of Ben and Eddie

Roald Dahl Museum and Story Centre
81-83 High Street
Great Missenden
HP16 0AL
(01494) 892192
admin@roalddahlmuseum.org
www.roalddahlmuseum.org

'This museum is in Buckinghamshire, about an hour from Guildford. It's a bit of a drive but we did it one Sunday afternoon, stopping off for lunch on the way, and it didn't seem too far to go at all.

I would describe it as quite a 'new concept' museum and it was certainly like nothing I'd ever visited before. It's quite small, really only three rooms and a corridor, but in each room you are bombarded with information and inspiration from every direction, as it's all projected on to floors, ceilings and walls. There are soundtracks to listen to, books to look through, activities to do, interactive displays to study… The longer you wander around each room the more you discover and absorb. Because it is quite small, too many people would spoil the experience, so you are allocated timed tickets that are easier to book online.

Although the museum gives you a fairly full history of Dahl's life, its aim seems more to encourage children to understand his joy of writing and to inspire them to do the same. When you arrive, each child is given a little 'inspirations book' and pencil to jot down ideas for stories and characters. The final room, which my children absolutely loved, was purely designed to inspire writing. There were *loads* of really imaginative activities to get the children thinking creatively and enjoying language.

The museum also runs some great workshops based on themes from Dahl's books. During our visit, there was a chocolate-decorating workshop inspired by *Charlie and Chocolate Factory*. If you have children who enjoy Roald Dahl stories or like writing their own then they would love this place and younger siblings brought along for the ride would have enough to entertain them too.'

Jo, mum of Thomas, George and Rebecca

Science Museum
Exhibition Road
South Kensington
SW7 2DD
(0870) 870 4868
www.sciencemuseum.org.uk

'The Discovery area of the *Science Museum* is superb and you can quite easily while away a day here. There are great interactive learning experiences for the young, and these range in difficulty so will challenge older siblings too. Of course, there is the rest of the Science Museum too, which boys in particular find very interesting.

I would suggest that you either take your own 'picnic' (an area is designated for this) or eat elsewhere (although there are two cafés).'

Debra, mum of Ben and Eddie

V&A Museum of Childhood
Cambridge Heath Road
Bethnal Green
E2 9PA
(020) 8983 5200
www.vam.ac.uk/moc

'This is a lovely old-fashioned museum that has been completely renovated with glass cabinets displaying all sorts of old toys and games that will bring back lots of memories. There are a few hands-on exhibits and usually some travelling exhibitions going on where children can get involved in art activities, workshops, treasure hunts etc., but for the most part it is just looking and admiring.

It is a large airy space with plenty of room for running around and there is a café in the middle of the ground floor serving great food for parents but not much basic fare for children. Probably aimed more at the older child although my four-year-old was happy to gaze admiringly at the cabinets of old Star Wars figures for hours!'

Bridget, mum of Jessie and Luke

Places to Visit

Weald & Downland Open Air Museum
Singleton
Chichester
PO18 0EU
(01243) 811363
office@wealddown.co.uk
www.wealddown.co.uk

'A pleasant day trip, set in gentle countryside with plenty to see; children particularly love the rare breeds of [farm livestock] and heavy horses. It is seldom crowded and makes a great place to wander around in good weather. Our favourite part is visiting the working Lurgashall watermill where you can buy bags of grain for feeding the ducks and enormous carp in the lake.

There is a simple restaurant and plenty of space for picnicking. A relaxing day out.'
Emma, mum of Conrad and Imogen

Theme Parks

Chessington World of Adventures
Leatherhead Road
KT9 2NE
(0870) 999 0045
www.chessington.co.uk
[Put 'parent and toddler club' into the search on the Chessington website, and find parent and toddler admission vouchers for £11.00 (2007) including a free coffee.]

'We had a great day out here when my son was two and a half. He was short enough to get in free, but was tall enough to go on some of the rides. He loved the log flume and runaway train roller coaster. Although it's worth going slightly out of season to avoid long queues, Chessington has a scheme whereby one adult can go on a ride [after initially queuing] while the other looks after the children, and then as soon as the first adult is off the ride, the second can go on straightaway without having to queue.'
Louise, mum of Joseph and Emilia

Legoland
Winkfield Road
Windsor
SL4 4AY
(08705) 040404
visitorservices@legoland.co.uk
www.legoland.co.uk
[*Tesco* clubcard vouchers can be exchanged for *Legoland* entry tickets and/or annual pass. See www.tesco.com/clubcard/deals for details.]

'*Legoland* makes me wish I'd been born thirty years later. My son says it's the "best place in the world" and if I were four I'd probably agree. The rides are very good; although I imagine once children get into double digits (years-wise) they may find it a bit childish! Take a towel/change of clothes as it's easy to get wet! But there is a lot on offer including puppet and adventure shows. It's pretty tiring and guarantees a good night's sleep afterwards (I think that goes for the kids too).

Queuing is the one big downside, so brave the colder midweek days and avoid

Places to Visit

weekends and holidays. My son and I went once on a drizzly midweek day in May and virtually had the place to ourselves! (although note that it is sometimes shut on Tuesdays and Wednesdays outside of peak season).

I recommend taking your own food as the on-site fare is limited and only adds to the cost. As a one-off it's expensive and some of the more exciting rides are at additional cost. An annual pass pays for itself after three or four trips.'
David, dad of Harry

Paultons Park
Ower, nr. Romsey
SO51 6AL
(023) 8081 4442
www.paultonspark.co.uk

'This is a real favourite of ours. It takes about an hour to get there from Guildford. It's a theme park specifically designed for the little ones. There are loads of rides including water slides, mini roller coasters, carousels, plus walk-through areas setting out nursery rhyme tales and *Toad of Toad Hall*, as well as trampolines and a bouncy castle. All the little sit-on rides that you find outside Sainsbury's etc. are free and when my two-year-old can't go on a ride with his brother he loves to go for a ride with *Winnie the Pooh, Postman Pat, Thomas* etc. There are only two rides that you need to be over 110cm for, the rest are 90cm or under. There is also a fantastic grotto there at Christmas.' [See 'Seasonal Events'.]
Sarah, mum of Zack and Fin

Trains, Cars and Aeroplanes

Bluebell Railway
Sheffield Park Station
TN22 3QL
(01825) 720825 (timetables)
info@bluebell-railway.co.uk
www.bluebell-railway.co.uk

'This steam-hauled passenger railway line is based in East Sussex. The line can be joined at either Sheffield Park Station, nr East Grinstead (best location) or via Horsted Keynes. You have the option to travel on the trains or simply buy a platform ticket where you can watch the steam trains, signals and operating practices of an old country branch line. Seasonal events include the Easter Eggstravaganza, Santa Express and Days Out with Thomas. A café and baby-changing facilities are available at the stations. *Sheffield Gardens*, which is free for *RHS Wisley* cardholders, is close to Sheffield Park Station, so combined with the Bluebell line, it makes for a great day out.'
Jo, mum of Oliver and Jake

Brands Hatch Circuit
Fawkham
Longfield
DA3 8NG
(01474) 872331
www.motorsportvision.co.uk

'Only a 50-minute drive from Guildford, *Brands Hatch* is an exciting day out for dads and sons alike. Most weekends have

some event going on. *Brands Hatch* is good for families; there is a small playground and a restaurant, and a large grassy bank where you can park the car and have a picnic while watching the cars from a safe distance. It's not too noisy for little ears, and the circuit is built in a small valley providing a good view of the track from most spectator points.'
Brendan, dad of Winston and Harvey

Fairoaks Airport
Chobham
GU24 8HU
(01276) 857700
info@alanmann.co.uk
www.alanmann.co.uk

'The airport is mainly used by small private planes and helicopters and is a great place to watch them taking off and landing. The *Hangar Café*, located within the flight centre serves great coffees and muffins, as well as sandwiches and hot lunches and is a good place to pass an hour on a rainy day. The restaurant also has an outside area where you can get really close to the planes…can get a bit noisy sometimes though!'
Marguerite, mum of David and Dylan

Guildford Train Station
Station Approach
GU1 4UT
(0845) 600 0650

'This may not sound like a very promising 'Place to Visit' but it's been a lifesaver at times when we're going stir-crazy at home. My train-obsessed toddler loves to go onto the platforms and watch the trains coming and going and the signal lights changing colour. With him safely strapped into his buggy, I've been known to sit for a while on Platform 2, having a nice cup of coffee and a flapjack, while he chats to me about what's going on and the baby sleeps in the sling. You sometimes need to get a (free) platform ticket, but the staff are very understanding of toddler train-spotting habits and never seem to mind how long we stay.'
Jo, mum of James and Daisy

Mercedes-Benz World
Brooklands Drive
Weybridge
KT13 0SL
(0870) 400 4000
mbworld@mercedes.co.uk
www2.mercedes-benz.co.uk
[Also see review for Brooklands Museum earlier in this chapter.]

'We strayed into *Mercedes-Benz World* on a very wet day when we had intended to go to *Brooklands Museum*. On the same site as *Brooklands*, *Mercedes-Benz World* is like a huge car showroom where no one minds if little feet climb all over the expensive upholstery. My five-year-old had a great time pretending to drive, watching the 'skid pan' and sitting in the sports cars. There is a nice café, a baby-change area, a crèche, which we didn't use but which looked well set up and best of all it's free. No one tried to sell us a car either!'
Julie, mum of Ben and Katie

Places to Visit

Watercress Line
The Railway Station
Alresford
SO24 9JG
(01962) 733810
info@watercressline.co.uk
www.watercressline.co.uk
[See also Day Out with Thomas later in this chapter.]

'This is an excellent and highly recommended day out. Visitors of all ages can savour the unique sights, sounds and smells of steam travel on a scenic journey through 10 miles of beautiful countryside between Alton and Alresford. It took us about 20 minutes to get to Alton from Guildford and we had a superb day out. The fact it was also Mother's Day [2007] made it even more special. The tickets were £10.00 per adult, and £5.00 for over-twos. This was for a return journey but you can hop on and off at the stations in between (Ropley, Medstead). Ropley has a picnic area and small play area, and in the summer is excellent for sitting on the grass watching the trains chuff past. Ella loved sitting in the old-style carriages and was chuffing away to the sound of the train! Visit the website for special events held throughout the year and the seasonal timetable.'
Lynn and Paul, parents of Ella

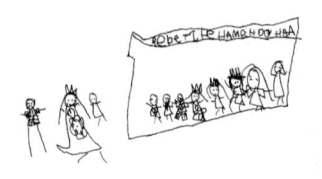

Other Days Out

London Eye
Westminster Bridge Road
SE1 7PB
(0870) 990 8883
customer.services@ba-londoneye.com
www.londoneye.com

'The *London Eye* is easy to get to since it's within walking distance of Waterloo. It's best to go when the weather is clear. There's a great view of London and it travels slowly enough to really take in all the sights. You can also go after dark, if you want to see the city lit up. The kids loved to pick out all their favourite familiar London locations. I was a bit worried how they would feel about the height, but they weren't a bit concerned. There can be a bit of a queue during holiday times, but it seems to go fairly quickly. If you have a buggy, there is a place to park it as you aren't allowed to take it on. Overall, we thoroughly enjoyed it. The kids still talk about it a year later. It's not cheap though; adults £14.50, children £7.25, under-fives free.'
Vonda, mum of Thomas

Gunwharf Quays Outlet Village
Gunwharf Quays
Portsmouth
PO1 3TZ
(023) 9283 6700
gwq-info@landsecurities.com
www.gunwharf-quays.com

'This is a retail outlet village in the heart of the Portsmouth Docks. As well as shopping for clothes in stores like *Gap*, *Fat Face*, *Clarks*, *M&S* and *Next*, there are also other sights to see that make it a full day out, that I would rate as really good.

About an hour's drive from Guildford, you drive through Portsmouth to get to the Quays. There is lots of parking and the lift brings you into a small square, which has a few children's activities like a carousel, small train and trampoline. While the rides are a bit expensive, they do give you an option when your toddler gets bored of shopping. There are many places to eat ranging from *Pizza Express* to *Bar 38*. We ate at *Tootsies*, an American bar and grill and the staff were happy to warm food for our twin babies, and had a good children's menu for our toddler.

If you don't want to shop, you can just watch the ferries dock and exit (which mesmerised our three-year-old), and also visiting the famous Spinnaker Tower, a sail-shaped tower of 170 metres from which the view, on a good day, is fantastic. Great place for walking around with buggies, but some of the shops were a bit tight for a double buggy. Clean toilet and baby-changing facilities.'

Rena, mum of Holly, Thomas and Kate

Portsmouth Historic Dockyard
HM Naval Base,
PO1 3LJ
(023) 9283 9766
enquiries@historicdockyard.co.uk
www.historicdockyard.co.uk

'This is a great day out for slightly older children – our five-year-old loved it,
although so did our six-month-old baby. We drove, but you can also get there by train (to Portsmouth Harbour), which would add to the excitement. The Dockyard contains *HMS Victory*, the *Mary Rose* and lots of interactive exhibits bringing naval history to life. There is also a harbour tour by boat that takes in great views of aircraft carriers and war ships anchored in the harbour. A trip to *Gunwharf Quays* (see p100) and the *Spinnaker Tower* is also easily possible from here.'

Julie, mum of Ben and Katie

Seasonal Events – Spring

Surrey County Show
Held at Stoke Park
8 Birtley Courtyard (for contact)
Bramley
GU5 0LA
(01483) 890810
scas@surreycountyshow.co.uk
www.surreycountyshow.co.uk
[Usually held on the second May Bank Holiday.]

'The County Show is great fun, and a tradition in our family. There is plenty to see and do (and eat!), and it is always sunny (well, has been lately!) It's not a cheap day out, but if you're in the market for some farm food and have nothing else to do that day, it won't disappoint.'

Paige, mum of Miranda and Leo

'We went when Maia was only 18 months; we enjoyed looking at all the animals and

Places to Visit

other displays and will definitely go again when she is older (when it might be more suited to her). It is expensive to get in, so go on a sunny day and stay all day to make the most of it! I would recommend that you go with children that don't need a buggy, as it was quite hard going when we went – the rain didn't help.'
Jude, mum of Maia

Seasonal Events – Spring/Summer

Day out with Thomas
The Watercress Line
Ropley Station
Station Hill
SO24 0BL
(01962) 733810
info@watercressline.co.uk
www.watercressline.co.uk
[Thomas Days Out run for about ten days during Easter and in August each year.]

'Get to see the real Thomas, Percy, Henry, James and Toad and Daisy the Diesel in the Hampshire countryside. You can get on at Alresford (a pretty village), Ropley or Alton Station.

Most of the action takes place at Ropley, including rides in a Diesel engine and a coach pulled by Thomas, and races between Thomas and Diesel overseen by the Fat Controller. There is also an inflatable bouncy slide/castle – although long queues can effectively mean your child often has time for only one go. There is also some kind of children's entertainer – in 2007 it was Punch & Judy. We didn't take a buggy as there is not much walking to do but you can put folded buggies on the trains in the brake coach [or leave with picnics in a designated marquee near the entrance at Ropley]. We took a picnic on the train – very civilised.'
Alex, dad of Dominic and Laura

'My boys always enjoy these. Your day ticket gives you unlimited travel on the trains, usually pulled by Henry and Daisy [from Alresford to Alton].

At Ropley, Thomas races against Diesel, and you can get rides a short way up and down the track with them. Also at Ropley there is a giant bouncy slide (though children do have to be big enough to climb up the bouncy steps on their own) and regular entertainment from Mr Wizard [or 'Punch & Judy']. You can visit the engine sheds and see James who is not well at the moment. Sometimes you can climb up onto his footplate and pretend to be the driver.

Percy is at Alresford giving rides along to the sidings and back. Also at Alresford, there is usually Bulgy the bus and a traction engine. For refreshments there is the usual station buffet at Alresford and a variety of vans selling food and drink at Ropley. There are shops selling all sorts of Thomas merchandise at Alresford, Ropley and Alton. All these stations have toilets and changing facilities. We can easily spend the whole day here and still not manage to do all the things on offer.'
Kay, mum of Alex, Brian and Theo.

Seasonal Events – Summer

All Saints Church Summer Fete
Onslow Village
GU2 7QJ
(01483) 572006
info@allsaintschurchgfd.org.uk
www.allsaintschurchgfd.org.uk

'If you live in the Onslow Village area and have young children, then this is an event to look out for. It is usually held over lunchtime, one Saturday in June. It's a real community event, with all the usual stalls, a bouncy castle and a barbecue well-stocked from the local butcher. The book, toy and plant stalls are always favourites and we always love watching the dancing display by the local ballet school.'
Jo, mum of Thomas, George and Rebecca

Annual Raft Race
Millmead
(07719) 695714
vicquayle@aol.com
www.guildfordlions.co.uk

'The first Saturday in July (see the local paper) usually marks the start of the Guildford Festival and the Annual Raft Race. All manner of local community groups and companies enter rafts ranging from engineering masterpieces to vessels that would be lucky to reach the start line! Rafts begin gathering by Millmead lock a couple of hours before the start time, and we often have fun wandering around them. However, our favourite position for watching is on the pedestrian bridge by the cinema. The flour throwing and water squirting antics are usually well under way and one or two rafts have usually started disintegrating which adds to the amusement.'
Jo, mum of Thomas, George and Rebecca

Model Steam Rally (GMES)
Guildford Model Engineering Society Ltd
London Road
GU1 1TU
secretary@gmes.org.uk (Subject: GMES)
www.gmes.org.uk

'There is an unusual attraction tucked away in the far end of Stoke Park – the GMES. The Society runs several open days during the spring and summer (check out the website for dates), and there is a lot to see: model trains, scaled-down trains you can ride on, exhibitions, stalls and refreshments. The charity days have a country fair atmosphere!'
Sonya, mum of Eleanor and Charles

'This is great fun. It is held over a weekend some time in July at Stoke Park. There are model railways, aeroplane engines, model traction engines, exhibition stands and boating lakes. For a small charge, you can go on steam train rides. There are stands selling all sorts of things and refreshments. Children get in for free, so it can be a good value event.'
Kay, mum of Alex, Brian and Theo.

'We love the open days held about once a month here in the summer. There are loads of steam and a few electric trains to

ride on. The trains don't travel too fast. There are two different tracks to go on. You buy tickets (50p per ride) at the ticket office and have it punched by the ticket collector before the train departs. This all adds up to an exciting experience for train-mad youngsters. There are smaller models inside the building and by the engine sheds. On charity days there are stalls, games and bouncy castles.'
Sally, mum of James

Seasonal Events – Autumn

Guildford Book Festival
(01483) 444334
www.guildfordbookfestival.co.uk

'The Guildford Book Festival (held during October half term) has really established itself in recent years, and has an excellent range of speakers, readers and events. There are always a good number of children's events, including some for very young children.'
Victoria, mum of Catherine

Wizard Week at the Watercress Line
The Watercress Line
The Railway Station
Alresford
SO24 9JG
(01962) 733810
info@watercressline.co.uk
www.watercressline.co.uk

'This runs during October half-term. The trains and stations are decorated with spooky things. The staff are all dressed up and enter into the spirit of the event. They give out goodie bags on the trains containing Halloween toys and jokes. There are various Halloween-themed activities, such as broom-making, owls and magic shows. This is a good fun event.'
Kay, mum of Alex, Brian and Theo

Seasonal Events – Winter

Fireworks Night
All Saints Church
Onslow Village
GU2 7QJ
(01483) 572006
info@allsaintschurchgfd.org.uk
www.allsaintschurchgfd.org.uk

'This fireworks show is lovely; it's really family-oriented, and is held early enough in the evening for all the kids to enjoy.'
Paige, mum of Miranda and Leo

Switching on the Christmas lights
Guildford High Street

'This usually happens on the last Thursday in November at about 7.00 pm. For our family it has become a real Christmas tradition. We love the atmosphere and the feeling of community spirit as we all gather under the clock ready for the countdown. The *Salvation Army* Band is always there, as are a whole range of street-sellers with their candy floss, roast chestnuts, hot dogs and things that glow! In recent years, the switching on of the lights has been followed by fireworks from the top of White Lion Walk.

Another tradition worth knowing about (although how long it will continue I don't know!) is that *'Heals'* in Tunsgate stays open extra late and offers free drinks and snacks (fruit cake, sweets etc.) The staff bravely allow people to take over their furniture department, encouraging people to relax on their very expensive sofas and armchairs while sipping their wine and eating their chocolates. They even lay on live music!'
Jo, mum of Thomas, George and Rebecca

Father Christmas at Bocketts Farm
Young Street
Fetcham
Leatherhead
KT22 9BS
(01372) 363764
www.bockettsfarm.co.uk

'For a really fabulous experience to see Father Christmas go to *Bocketts Farm*. It's not exactly cheap but you don't have to pay for entry to the farm itself and you come away with a decent toy (usually soft). The visit starts at the entry gate where you climb into the mini trailer, which takes you to Father Christmas' grotto. Mum and dad can walk alongside if the little one is nervous and you disembark at the barn. You walk through the hay-bale lined barn, through the 'toy preparation area' to Father Christmas himself who is thoroughly unthreatening.

I have never seen any child in tears or fearful, instead you see children with wide, excited eyes, desperate to tell him what they want for Christmas. An enchanting visit and one we as parents look forward to as much as our children! Sensible family toilets and changing tables next to the barn.'
Sonya, mum of Eleanor and Charles

Father Christmas at Paultons Park
Ower, nr. Romsey
SO51 6AL
(023) 8081 4442
www.paultonspark.co.uk

'This is a real favourite of ours. There is a fantastic grotto there at Christmas that you walk through before getting to see the man himself. Presents are always very well chosen by Father Christmas! All the rides within the park are open. We have visited at Christmas time for the past few years and there have been no queues for any of the rides and we have been lucky enough to have dry days.'
Sarah, mum of Zack and Fin

Christmas Services at All Saints' Church
All Saints' Church
Onslow Village
GU2 7QJ
(01483) 572006
info@allsaintschurchgfd.org.uk
www.allsaintschurchgfd.org.uk

'*All Saints' Church* in Onslow Village is very child-friendly. At Christmas there is a very welcoming carol service, a Christingle service, and a children's nativity on Christmas Eve. The nativity is very visual and even young children love

Places to Visit

it. The vicar is extremely welcoming and it doesn't matter if your child runs around and causes a bit of chaos!'
Liz, mother of Isabelle and Evie

St Saviour's Christingle service
Woodbridge Road
GU1 4QD
(01483) 455333
office@st-saviours.org.uk
www.st-saviours.org.uk

'Christingle usually happens mid-afternoon on Christmas Eve although can vary depending upon where in the week Christmas falls. It is a short, very child-centred service, during which the children make/receive a Christingle and it gives us all a quiet moment to remember the other side of Christmas.

Many other churches have similar Christingle or Crib services around this time so look out for one in your local church.'
Jo, mum of Thomas, George and Rebecca

Astolat Model Railway Circle Exhibition
Guildford Methodist Church
Woodbridge Road
GU1 4RG
(01483) 235387 (Vic Langston)
www.astolatmrc.co.uk

'This is on the third Saturday in January at the Methodist Hall on Woodbridge Road. My train-mad boys always enjoy this. There are lots of model railway layouts to see of different styles and gauges. There are also one or two where you can take a turn to control the trains. The refreshments stall usually has a variety of home-made cakes.'
Kay, mum of Alex, Brian and Theo

Playgrounds

Playgrounds – what would we do without them? They are a simple and failsafe option on a day when you just have to get out of the house, or could be a great day out if combined with a picnic and a walk. Listed below are as many playgrounds as we could find in Guildford and surrounding areas, plus one or two extra, where it's worth making the extra effort to go those extra few miles to get there.

Guildford Borough Council has a page on its website dedicated to playgrounds. *http://www.guildford.gov.uk/guildfordweb/leisure/parkscountryside/parks/playgrounds.htm* Some of its information is echoed below, but do read on to get a good idea of what people think of them!

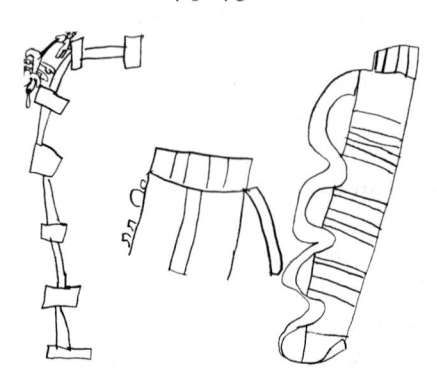

Abinger Hammer playground
A25 Guildford – Dorking
[See also 'Duck feeding and Paddling' review for Abinger Hammer earlier in this chapter.]

'Play on the climbing frame in the corner of the cricket pitch. If you need a picnic you can stop first at Kingfisher Farm Shop next to the cricket pitch, or cross over the road to the tea shop.'
Sonya, mum of Eleanor and Charles

Artillery Road playground
Stoke Fields
[Suitable for toddlers and juniors; 2 items of equipment.]

Baird Drive playground
Wood Street Village
[Suitable for toddlers and juniors; 4 items of equipment.]

Bannisters Field playground
Egerton Road (by Tesco)
[Suitable for toddlers; 2 items of equipment.]

Barnwood Road playground
Park Barn
[Suitable for toddlers and juniors; 4 items of equipment.]

Broadwater Park
Summers Lane
Godalming
(Two car parks: Godalming Leisure Centre and Off Nursery Road)
[Park undergoing full reconstruction at time of publication, so the playground might well end up being different to that detailed below.]

'This is a great park, with the added bonus of having a nice-sized sandpit, a boat-shaped climbing frame and tunnels, as well as the usual swings. There is also a lake nearby to walk around with lots of ducks, geese and swans (the swans can be a little too keen for food), toilets and a car park. Can be a little exposed on a windy day.'
Jacqui, mum of Harry and Megan

'Ducks, great playground and sandpit, recreation ground, walk around the lake.'
Paige, mum of Miranda and Leo

Bushy Hill Drive playground
Merrow
[Suitable for toddlers and juniors; 6 items of equipment.]

Derby Road playground
Park Barn
[Suitable for toddlers and juniors; 5 items of equipment.]

Devoil Close playground
Weybrook Park
Burpham
[Suitable for toddlers; 3 items of equipment.]

'This small playground is ideal for toddlers. It has a toddler swing and a small climbing frame with slide and fireman's pole. Because it is not on a

Places to Visit

main road, you usually have the park to yourself.'
Louise, mum of Joseph and Emilia

Diana, Princess of Wales' Memorial Playground
Kensington Gardens
W2 2UH
(020) 7298 2141
kensington@royalparks.gsi.gov.uk
www.royalparks.gov.uk/parks/ kensington_gardens/diana_playground. cfm

'This playground has a wooden pirate ship surrounded by more sand than on a normal beach. Kids can play inside the large galleon, dig with diggers in the sand and climb the masts. In addition, there is a water-play area (operates in warmer months), which kids young and old love (take a change of clothes and a bucket or containers for them to fill), walks through teepees, a raised wooden walk through trees, slides and swings, musical chimes they can play, etc. It is brilliantly designed, and on a nice day, this is probably my favourite place for the kids in London (how many times have I been dragged here?!?)

Toilet facilities are modern and clean, and there is a café although many people take picnics. Afterwards the children can take a walk (or bike ride, which is permitted here) down to the lake, visit the fountains to the east, or look at all the artwork and paintings that hang from the railings along Bayswater Road. A definite thumbs up!

You can access the playground from the far North-west side of the park, from Bayswater Road.'
Debra, mum of Ben and Eddie

Foxenden Quarry playground
York Road
[Suitable for juniors; 4 items of equipment.]

Fairlands playground
On the corner of Fairlands Avenue and Brocks Lane
[Suitable for toddlers; 4 items of play equipment.]

'This playground is located behind the community centre and beside the GP surgery. It is generally clean and tidy, but while it does not have much for smaller babies or toddlers, it does have a safe baby swing.'
Heather, mum of Jessica

Glendale Drive playground
Burpham
[Suitable for toddlers and juniors; 3 items of equipment.]

Godalming playground
Behind Crown Court carpark

'Our favourite playground. It has a small wooden climbing frame for toddlers and a larger one for when they get a little older and more adventurous. The toddler swings are a bit creaky but there is more than enough other apparatus to make up for this.

We usually like to combine a trip here with a walk along the river to feed the ducks.

The car park is just over the road.'
Jacqui, mum of Harry and Megan

Gomshall playground
A25 Guildford – Dorking

'This one is a well-kept secret, and certainly worth visiting! All the equipment is wooden, and there are some unusual pieces, which make it a treat to visit. The equipment caters for younger children too, and it is adjacent to a big field for running and ball-playing. We've brought a picnic here in the summer, and it was glorious! Worth noting, however, that there are no toilets.

It is off the A25 (drive towards Dorking, turn right just before *Blubeckers*, go past the car park, and it's your next right).'
Kris, mum of Olivia and Victoria

'Take the little lane, over the bridge, next to *The Mill at Gomshall*, which leads towards the village green. Here is a small car park and a pretty all-wood playground. It has some unusual apparatus that the kids love. It can be combined with lunch at *Blubeckers* (see review under *Eating Out*).'
Debra, mum of Ben and Eddie

Kings College playground
Southway
Park Barn
[Suitable for juniors; 6 items of equipment.]

Kingston Meadows playground
Kingston Avenue
East Horsley

'This park was re-opened last summer with brand new equipment. The park is split into two areas – toddler equipment and older children's climbing frames. There are secure gates around the park. There is a grass area, basketball net, and tennis courts for older children. There are toilets in the nearby village hall. A really safe environment to let the children run off some steam!'
Jane, mum of Jessica

'East Horsley play area is set in parkland behind the medical centre. Newly refurbished approximately 18 months ago, two areas, would suit children from toddlers to 11-year-olds. Lots of parking adjacent.'
Vicki, mum of George and Finlay

Onslow Village recreation ground and arboretum
Access from Powell Close, past the infant school, off Manor Way, and off Wilderness Road
[Suitable for toddlers and juniors; 6 items of play equipment.]

'This is a lovely little playground with swings, a climbing frame and slide, a seesaw and a springy horse and elephant to ride. It is a great trip to get us out of the house if we are going spare and can be tied in with a little walk around the arboretum, which is just next to it. The

playground, being next to the infant school, gets very busy in summer when the children come out of school, so if you have younger children it is best avoided from about 3.00 pm during term-time.'
Katherine, mum of Holly and Hazel

The Oval playground
Off The Chase
Guildford Park

'There is a lovely children's playground located off The Oval at the foot of the cathedral. It's set back off the road and in addition to the usual swings and climbing frames it also has a good bit of green space for ball games or kite flying. The only gripe is that there is often a fair bit of broken glass by the playing area. The council does seem to attempt to clear this up fairly regularly though. This park could do with a little loving care and updating of the apparatus.'
Jacqui, mum of Harry and Megan

Park Barn Drive playground
Park Barn
[Suitable for juniors; 3 items of equipment.]

Parson's Green playground
Slyfield
[Suitable for toddlers and juniors; 3 items of equipment.]

Stoke recreation ground
Recreation Road
[Suitable for toddlers and juniors; 10 items of equipment.]

'Good little playground for smaller children. The baby swings are lower than many and there's a rather clever roundabout as well as the usual climbing frame/slide. Watching the football on the recreation ground is a big hit too.'
Victoria, mum of Catherine

Send recreation ground
Send Road

'Two baby swings, four bigger swings, climbing frame and slide, bouncy sheep and triangle bouncer. Nearby is a coffee shop, post office, hairdresser, beautician, butcher, newsagent and a charity shop so you can do some useful bits of shopping in the same outing. Also picnic bench, basketball courts and large area for running and ball games.'
Beth, mum of Abigail

Shamley Green playground
Lords Hill

'Head out of Guildford towards Cranleigh on the B2128, and you'll pass through the picturesque village of Shamley Green. The village sports a fantastic pub (the *Red Lion*, child-friendly), village shop (ice creams and drinks for the purchasing thereof), cricket green and duck pond. It also has a playground, which is popular with locals, but as it's off the beaten track it's never overcrowded. It has a set of swings I can't prise my toddler away from, a set of 'big boy swings' (we have aspirations), a slide, rocking horse, seesaw, roundabout, climbing frame, wooden train, and a sort

of 'hammock' swing that slightly older children love to lay down full length in. There is also a picnic table. The area isn't fenced in, but it's located on a back road that sees very little traffic, and there are some lovely walks in the surrounding countryside. To find it, just before you enter Shamley Green turn right into 'Lords Hill', follow the road, and you'll see the playground on your right. If you miss the turning, carry on into the village, turn right past the village shop on the green, and carry straight on, past the entrance to Longacre school, following the road as it bends to the right, and the playground will be on your left.'
Rachel, mum of Felix and Phoebe

Shere playground
Upper Street
[See also 'Duck feeding and Paddling' entry earlier in this chapter.]

'Right next to a nursery and directly behind the village hall, this small, good old-fashioned playground has a big slide, climbing frame, swings and is near a large recreation ground for good old-fashioned run-arounds! Also near the village for tea, duck-feeding, etc.'
Paige, mum of Miranda and Leo

Stoke Park Gardens
Stoke Road
[Suitable for toddlers and juniors; 16 items of equipment.]

'This is my children's favourite park in Guildford, especially in the summer when you can spend several hours there. There are large grassed areas, formal gardens and picnic areas. Facilities range from a large, shallow splash pool with a springy rubber floor that is toddler-friendly but fun for bigger children too. The playground has a large climbing frame, an assault-course area to challenge the over-fours, swings and helter-skelter to name a few. Tennis courts and a putting green are also in the park, and there is a lake for model boats (bring your own!) and a kiosk with seating outside selling drinks, snacks and ice creams. The large car park shared with the college can be busy in the week, but parking is available on nearby roads.'
Rachel, mum of Amy, Thomas and Ella

'Chasing tennis balls on the courts is fun, even if just with the pushchair!'
Paige, mum of Miranda and Leo

'There's a wonderful paddling pool and ice cream kiosk, open from Easter. The playground is slightly more suited to older children.'
Kris, mum of Olivia and Victoria

Stoughton recreation park
Worplesdon Road
[Suitable for toddlers, juniors and teenagers; 7 items of equipment.]

'The park is located between Worplesdon Road, Aldershot Road, Northway and Fentum Road with access, via tarmac paths, from all but the Aldershot Road. The playground is situated at the bottom of the park under a couple of large oak

Places to Visit

trees. It has three separate activity enclosures suitable for toddlers, juniors and teenagers. It also has benches and tables for grown-ups to rest. It is generally litter free and visited on a regular basis by park rangers. This park is also practical for cycling practice and ball games for the family, except when it's used by the local football club for matches and practice.'
Nelly and Rhod, parents of Alys

'A really big open space that has a separate section with swings, climbing frames, slides, etc. The slides and other equipment are sectioned off according to age – so the really weenie ones can play on the baby swings without being bothered by the teenagers doing dunk shots in the basketball hoops! The grass park area seems to be well-kept, and very popular with youngsters on their bikes and playing ball games. The ground is also popular with dog walkers, but there are litter bins for their mess so it is really quite clean and attractive.'
Charlotte, mum of Karina

St Luke's playground
Warren Road

'Nice little playground, ideal if you're going to the doctor's surgery opposite. Two separate sections, one each for big and small children. Just slides and climbing frames plus a couple of bouncy animals/planes for the small ones. The small slide is particularly good – two straight ones side by side and a curvy one.'
Victoria, mum of Catherine

Sutherland Memorial Park
Clay Lane
Burpham

'This is a firm favourite of our family as it is easy to park at and can be combined with a shop or a drink at *Starbucks* in *Sainsbury's*! The playground is divided into two, with an area for toddlers with climbing frame, slides and baby swings. The older part is good fun with lots to sit on and a large climbing frame. In the summer, you can picnic in the park surrounding the play area. Possibly worth avoiding at 3.00 pm for half an hour due to Burpham school leavers!'
Rebecca, mum of Isabelle, Aimee and Robyn

'Fantastic location for bribing the little ones to behave on the trip round *Sainsbury's*! At the roundabout to the entrance to *Sainsbury's* is a good, well-maintained playground for a wide range of age groups. There is a separate, gated area for the younger ones, which I find useful, as older children can get a little careless with tots in all their excitement. In the summer there is usually an ice-cream van, which adds another dimension to the bribing option!'
Debra, mum of Ben and Eddie

'Fantastic playground with two separate play areas for younger and older children. Lots of variety for children of all ages. There's an adjacent grassy area for ball games/picnics. *Sainsbury's* (plus *Starbucks* coffee shop) is nearby for use of toilets.

It can get quite busy in the afternoons during term-time when children are leaving the local primary school. It is well looked after and always clean.'
Lisa, mum of Thomas

'Clean and safe. Two fenced in, main playgrounds for younger and older children, plus lots of space to run around and kick a ball. Gets busy at weekends, but enough equipment that kids don't have to wait too long to get their go. Favourite with Dads.'
Charlotte, mum of Noah

Tilehouse Open Space
Tarragon Drive
Also access from Angelica Road
[Suitable for toddlers – 5 items of play equipment, juniors – 3 big items of play equipment, and teenagers – 1 basketball area]

'This playground is situated close to the housing estate and approximately 200m from Worplesdon Road, which offers access via a tarmac path and across a grass field. The playground has a three separate activity enclosures suitable for toddlers, juniors and teenagers. The installations are different from those at Stoughton Recreation Park, which makes a nice change for children and parents who are in close enough proximity to choose between visits to either of these amenities. There is also a pond area where geese and ducks are often seen and appreciated by toddlers.'
Nelly and Rhod, parents of Alys

Waterside Road playground
Slyfield
[Suitable for toddlers and juniors, 6 items of equipment.]

West Clandon playground
The Street

'Tucked away at the back of the village hall in West Clandon, we discovered this little playground by chance. It has a lovely enclosed small toddler area with a climbing frame consisting of a small tunnel and slide, and also a larger enclosed grassy area with toddler swings and swings for older children, large seesaw and a very large slide! There's a bench to sit on and admire the view over the fields and there's a grassy area with a big tree for running around. There's usually plenty of parking at the side of the hall and it is usually pretty quiet.'
Marguerite, mum of David and Dylan

West Horsley playground
The Street

'This lovely playground has recently been renovated and is a great place to visit if you happen to be in the area, as it is about five miles from Guildford. It is located in a small grassy field beside the village hall with lots of parking available. There is a lovely wooden toddler climbing area with small slide, two toddler swings and swings for older children, a larger climbing frame with climbing net, slide and wobbly bridge, a small seesaw and a little roundabout. There is also a big hill

to run up and down, balancing beams to walk along and other climbing apparatus. Lots of tables and benches so great for a picnic. You can also play football in the middle of the playground and there is a basketball hoop for older children. It can get busy with older children after school.'
Marguerite, mum of David and Dylan

'Newly refurbished play area, very nice for the toddler and young school child. Fully enclosed area. Parking adjacent.'
Vicki, mum of George and Finlay

White House Lane playground
Off Jacob's Well Road

'This small playground is on our way home from *Sainsbury's* in Burpham, and if Sutherland Memorial Park has been passed but the moans from the back of the car haven't abated, this is a great place to stop off for a small boost of swings. There are toddler and big boy swings, plus a roundabout and a small climbing frame with a slide and a noisy metal tunnel to crawl through; there is also a duck pond close by, but the other side of the railings, so the ducks are safe from toddlers!'
Claire, mum of William

Woodside Road playground
Westborough
[Suitable for toddlers and juniors; 9 items of equipment]

Worplesdon Road playground
(Opposite Rosemary Crescent)

'This playground had a new separate toddler's area built at the beginning of this year (2007). There are two baby swings, a toddlers' climbing frame with slide and a roundabout in the new area. The existing area includes two swings, a slide and a climbing frame as well as a football/basketball area for older children. We go there at least twice a week and look at the ducks on the way past the pond.'
Nadine, mum of Noah and Luca

4

Public Transport

Kay, mum of Alex, Brian and Theo

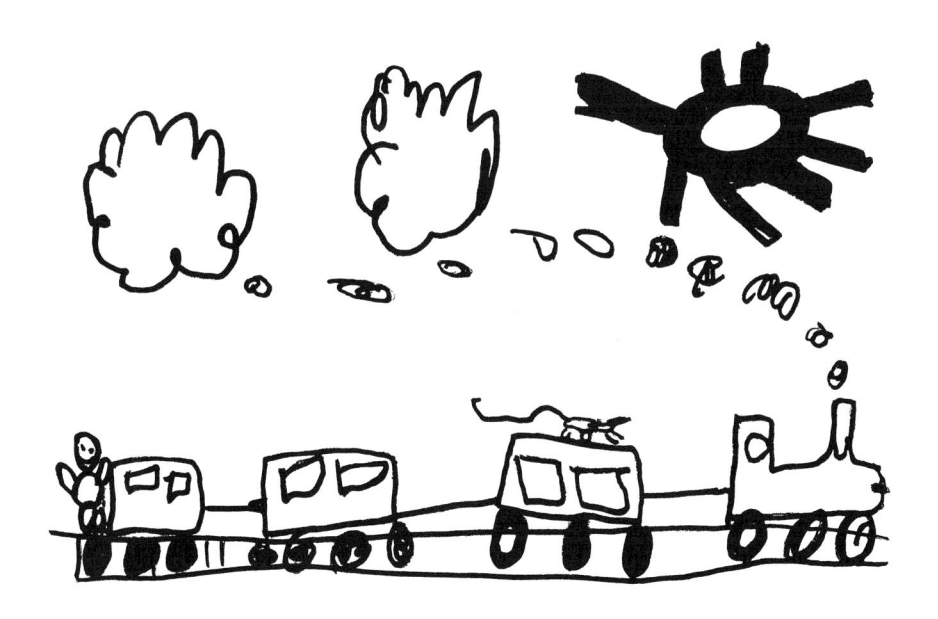

All the details for the places mentioned in this chapter can be found in *Things to Do* or *Places to Visit*.

Several bus routes are mentioned. You can find details for these at the travel office at the *Friary Bus Station*. *Traveline* will give you details of all public transport or you can contact the bus companies concerned:

Arriva	(01483) 505693	www.arriva.co.uk
Countryliner	(01483) 506919	www.countryliner-coaches.co.uk
Safeguard	(01483) 561103	www.safeguardcoaches.co.uk
Stagecoach	(0845) 1210180	www.stagecoachbus.com
Traveline	(0871) 2002233	www.traveline.org.uk
Traveline South	(0871) 2002233	www.travelinesoutheast.org.uk
Transport for London	(020) 7222 1234	www.tfl.gov.uk
Travel London	(01932) 745230	www.travellondonbus.co.uk

Using Public Transport

'I do not drive and so have no choice about using public transport. Where we go is influenced by what bus or train routes are available, but there are still plenty of places you can visit. Most trains and buses have low, wide doors these days, so getting on and off with a pushchair is not usually a problem, and there is usually space for you to park your buggy without having to fold it.

Going on public transport can have some advantages:

- It's more environmentally friendly
- There's no hassle about parking
- Children learn to be patient
- Some places (e.g. many *National Trust* locations) reward you if you arrive on public transport by giving you money off in the shop or café
- You learn to appreciate the things close by
- Days out can be more of an adventure
- You can interact with your children more on the journey by looking out for things or reading.

These are my favourite places to visit using public transport:

- **Guildford Spectrum Leisure Complex** [see *Things to Do*] – Swimming, skating, bowling and soft play. We seem to spend half our lives here. The 100 bus (*Arriva*) runs frequently from stop number 2 at Guildford bus station and is nearly always easy-access.

- **Wisley** [see p86] – The bus-stop is close to the entrance; I gather from those who drive that the car park can get very full. Bus 515 (*Travel London*) goes from stop 19 at Guildford bus station once an hour. You can also make use of the 'pram-walk' here.

- **Clandon Park** [see p74 & p79] – This is a *National Trust* site, so you can get vouchers for money off in the café or shop if you show your bus or train ticket at the entrance. The 463 (*Countryliner*) goes from stop 9 every two hours and stops very close to the entrance. Trains also run frequently to Clandon station but it is a reasonably long walk from there.

- **Stoke Park** [see p111] – Always lots to do. Numbers 3 (*Arriva* and *Safeguard* from stop 13 at the bus station), 34 and 35 (both *Arriva* from stop 6 at the bus station) go along Stoke Road, or you could go to London Road station on the train.

- **Sutherland Memorial Park** [see p112] – Play in the park and pop to *Sainsbury's*. The 36 (*Arriva*) runs every 20 minutes from stop 18 at the bus station. The 37 (*Arriva*) is the most direct route back.

- **Rokers Little Angels** [see p42] – My boys love this. The number 20 (*Stagecoach*) runs twice an hour from stop 14 at the bus station.

- **Claremont Landscape Gardens** [see p80] – This is a *National Trust* site, so you can get vouchers for money off in the café or shop if you show your bus ticket at the entrance. Bus 515 (*Travel London*) goes from stop 19 at Guildford

bus station once an hour. The bus stop is right by the entrance.
- **Watercress Line** [see p100 & p102] – For my train-mad boys, what could be better? Going on an electric train to get to the steam trains! Get the train towards Ascot and change at Aldershot for the Alton service.
- **Kew Gardens** [see p84] – We only did this recently but it was a great success. I am sure we will do it again. You need to get the train to Clapham Junction, then change for Kew Bridge.
- **London** [see p72 & p100] – *London Aquarium*, *London Eye*, *London Ducktours* and boat trips on the *Thames* are only a short walk from *Waterloo*.'

Kay, mum of Alex, Brian and Theo

Out and About with a Pushchair…

'As a result of the *Disability Discrimination* legislation, most shops now have lifts between floors so it is fairly easy to shop with wheels. In addition many places have doors for wheelchairs that are useful when you have a pram or a buggy. Sometimes you have to ask about access but often it is simply a case of looking out for wheelchair signs in order to find the step-free access. *House of Fraser* is particularly good as there are ramps on each floor.

Guildford itself is pretty good for step-free access. Although places like Milkhouse Gate are difficult with a pram (and the hills still make me puff), there are subways under most of the major roads and these all have ramps as well as steps.

Guildford Borough Council actually has a 'walking strategy' and a 'walking forum' to encourage more people to walk. There are details on the website along with some suggested walking routes – *www.guildford.gov.uk/GuildfordWeb/ Environment/Transport/Walking.htm*

…by Bus

I have found that most of the buses are very good as you can fit the pram into the area set aside for wheelchairs/ buggies and still (just about) have room to sit down. Most of the buses are also able to lower the floor by the door as you enter or leave which is a big help when the base of the pram is full of shopping! All of the bus-stops in the Friary are step-free.

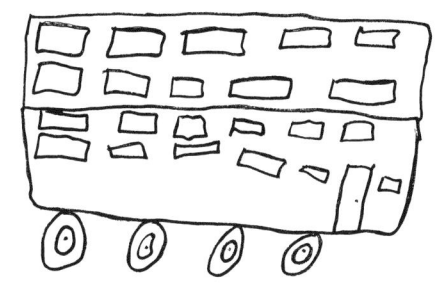

…by Train

Guildford is a useful station as the underpass means that all platforms have step-free access. Many other stations have lifts but these are often located behind the stairs and you may need to ask for them. *South West Trains* has a PDF map that you can download from its website (*www.southwesttrains.co.uk/SWTrains*). This shows all the stations with step-free access within its network and within the national rail network.

Similarly, *Transport for London* has PDF maps that include the tube, buses and tourist attractions (*www.tfl.gov.uk*). Access is not as good on the tube as it is on mainline trains, but I have found that people will usually help you to lift the pram up or down stairs if you smile at them nicely!

As regards the Guildford-London trains, I have found that the slow trains have more room for prams than the fast ones; however I think this is gradually changing as *South West Trains* seem to be using more commuter 'cattle truck' trains and fewer trains with narrow aisles.'
Katy, mum of Edward

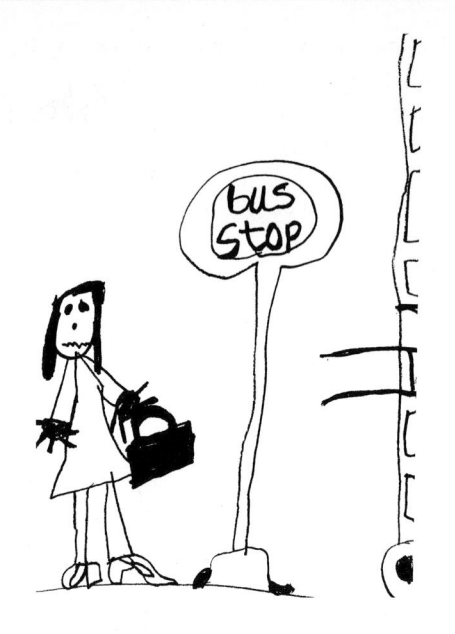

'The new trains with wheelchair spaces are great and my one-year-old loves going on the train. Even when there are no ramps at a station I've always found the staff immensely helpful.'
Victoria, mum of Catherine

5

Shopping

Jenny Kingston, mum of Imogen and Harrison
Liz Robinson, mum of Thomas

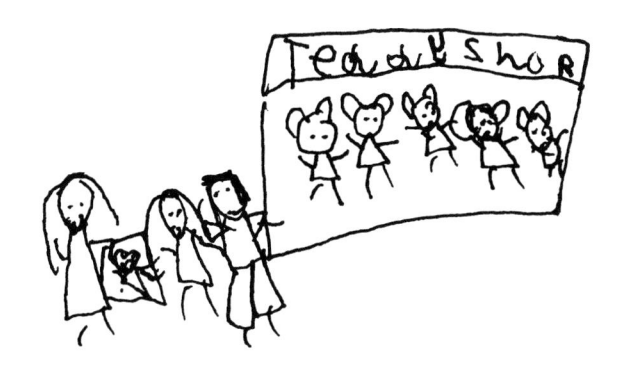

Whether you've just moved to the area or have lived here for many years, you often can't appreciate how very differently you come to rely on your town until you have little ones. The type of shops on your 'don't let me forget to go to...' list will often be more in the line of *Mothercare* and the *Early Learning Centre* than *Karen Millen* or *Monsoon*. However, take heart; this section will guide you through whether it's your first outing with a newborn or a quick trip in with older children.

Before we had children, my husband and I would often just wander into Guildford on a weekend to amble round the shops, grab some lunch in a café or a pub and catch a film before heading home. The town would always be full of families with buggies and kids in tow (often 20ft behind dragging their heels) and we would often wonder how they managed.

Now having two kids ourselves, we have learned to appreciate the wonders of Guildford from another level. Before children, we'd never ventured beyond *Debenhams*, but we now often walk down to *Millmead* to feed the many ducks and pigeons, or take a picnic to the top of the castle grounds where kids can

Shopping

run around and take a break from sitting in buggies. Although there aren't any playgrounds in town there are lots of shops, such as the *Early Learning Centre* and *The Disney Store*, where toys are set out for play. If you fancy a quick rest, *Costa* and *Starbucks* are very kid-friendly and will make 'babychinos' in little cups for your toddlers to feel like grown-ups.

Some weekends a quick trip to town does seem like a guided tour of every available public toilet, often requiring more than one visit, just to be sure!!! You quickly become an expert in knowing the nearest and easiest toilet to find from any given location in the high street, so do check out 'Public Toilets' at the end of this chapter. In addition to this, knowing the nearest place for food when the 'but I'm really very, very, very hungry/thirsty' wails commence, has become another very useful skill (see *Eating Out*).

Clothes

BHS
33 The Friary Centre
GU1 4YR
(01483) 8410193
www.bhs.co.uk

'BHS carries a relatively small range of baby and toddler clothes, but seems good for school uniforms. More importantly there are great toilets with both disabled and changing facilities at the rear left-hand side of the shop.'
Jenny, mum of Imogen and Harrison

Debenhams
Millbrook
GU1 3UU
(0844) 5616161
www.debenhams.com

'Debenhams stocks a number of clothing ranges including the lesser expensive own-brand range to the pricier *Designers at Debenhams* ranges by *Jasper Conran* (*j junior*) and *John Rocha* (*Rocha.little rocha*). The clothes always look good, are good quality and wear well. The *Early Learning Centre* toy department is right next to the clothing range on the first floor, and the restaurant, which is extremely baby and child friendly, is on the ground floor. The baby changing facilities are good too. Some of the changing rooms accommodate buggies, so it is possible for you to try on clothes while shopping with a child in a pushchair.'
Lisa, mum of Thomas

'This department store is great for trendy children's clothing and some designer ranges. You can also use your *Nectar* points (that you can gather by the bucket-load in *Sainsbury*'s) against your purchases. There is a large range of wedding apparel and accessories in spring. There is also an *Early Learning Centre* department adjacent to the children's clothing and a new area selling stylish baby equipment à la *White Company* style.'
Sonya, mum of Eleanor and Charles

120

Shopping

Gap Kids
68 High Street
GU1 3ES
(01483) 302959
www.gap.com

'This is our favourite shop for children's clothes in Guildford as it has trendy clothes that are very well made. The staff are always very helpful and give you hassle-free returns if you have bought clothes in the wrong size, for the wrong season, or that just don't suit. There is also a small play area.'
Nadine, mum of Noah and Luca

House of Fraser
105-111 High Street
GU1 3DU
(0870) 160 7245
www.houseoffraser.co.uk

'There is a small section of children's clothing on the first floor. Ranges like *Ralph Lauren*, *Elle*, *Timberland* and other designer ranges, as well as *House of Fraser*'s own. This section is next to the toilets and a single baby changing/feeding room. If this room is occupied you can end up waiting for a while. But then if you don't mind the wait, you can have a coffee in the coffee shop adjacent.'
Sonya, mum of Eleanor and Charles

'Takes a bit of working out, but when you know where the ramps are, *House of Fraser* is an easily navigable shop with wide aisles and efficient lifts.'
Charlotte, mum of Noah

Kontinental Kids
Level 2
The Friary Centre
North Street
GU1 4YT
(01483) 454343

'Not cheap, but a stylish addition to the Friary, selling French and Italian children's and babies' clothes.'
Victoria, mum of Catherine

Marks & Spencer
61-65 High Street
GU1 3EB
(01483) 502420
www.marksandspencer.com

'Good quality children's clothing. In my experience sizes tend to be larger than other makes – except for tights, which are smaller. They wash and wear and wear and wear. School clothing is very good quality – if you can imagine ever having a child old enough for school!'
Sonya, mum of Eleanor and Charles

'The shop is very buggy friendly with a great sized lift to gain access to all floors. The baby changing/disabled toilet is very good and it is nice and clean. It is a great size with a stool to sit on when breast feeding. The only down side is that it does get used a lot and therefore the few times I have used it to change Jessica and also to feed her I have felt I needed to hurry up because I could hear people outside waiting to use it.'
Linda, mum of Jessica

Shopping

'I was invited to use one of the fitting rooms to feed my baby, which is apparently something *M&S* offers.'
Tessa, mum of Daisy, Zach and Jake

'I sometimes seem to spend my life in *Marks & Spencer*'s roomy lift as I divide my time between children's clothes upstairs and food in the basement. There's a big disabled toilet/baby changing room on the first floor and you can get a single pushchair into any of the ordinary cubicles. I've fed Catherine on one of the many chairs dotted about peaceful corners of the store.'
Victoria, mum of Catherine

Millets
21 Friary Street
GU1 4EH
(01483) 573476
www.millets.co.uk

'Excellent children's outdoor gear, good prices, very knowledgeable and patient staff!'
Kris, mum of Olivia and Victoria

Monsoon/Accessorize
50-54 High Street
GU1 3ES
(01483) 572456
www.monsoon.co.uk

'*Monsoon* sells lovely babies and children's clothes. However there are always more clothes for little girls than for little boys. I always enjoy looking though. The children's department is in the first floor of the newly opened branch and there is even a lift.'
Nadine, mum of Noah and Luca

Next
1-2 White Lion Walk
GU1 3DN
(0870) 386 5166
www.next.co.uk
[Note: The children's department has recently expanded and moved to the first floor at the rear left-hand side behind the men's department, leaving a bit more space to manoeuvre a pushchair].

'The clothes from *Next* are excellent quality, look lovely, and I would say, are probably priced in the mid-range.'
Lisa, mum of Thomas

'Great children's clothing up to age five for both boys and girls. After five for the girls, I find that with a range that covers three to16 some clothes are way too adult in style for a five-year-old. However, if you hunt you can still find fairy T-shirts and frilly, girly skirts. It's not a huge range within the store for any of the age ranges

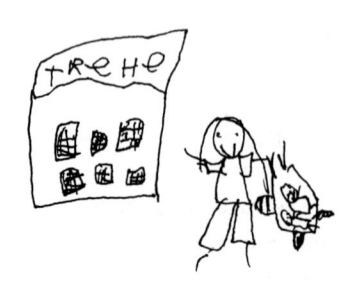

but if you get the catalogue the choice is vast.'
Sonya, mum of Eleanor and Charles

Primark
The Peacocks Centre
Woking
GU21 6GD
(01483) 720816
www.primark.co.uk

'Cheap essentials cannot be beaten on price. Larger sized clothes make good maternity wear.'
Lisa, mum of Lewis, Scarlett, Dylan, Saffron, Jude, and Reuben

'Set on the upper level in the *Peacocks Centre*, which is not that accessible with a pushchair due to high demand on the centre's lifts, it's a hot busy store any time of year! Staff are not the friendliest but you can get some great bargains if you are prepared to brave the negatives. Worth going once a quarter to stock up on vests and babygros, and basics, also great for cheap fashion whilst you are at your 'in between' sizes.'
Vicki, mum of George and Finlay

Stars
16 North Street
GU1 4AF
(01483) 306556

'*Stars* is a small boutique for babies and children selling designer brands, and holding smart, pretty stock. Not the cheapest, but good quality things. Worth a visit for a special occasion when you need to go that extra mile for something special. Look out for sales.'
Emma, mum of Charlotte and Louis

Trotters
Unit 6 White Lion Walk
GU1 3DN
(01483) 454668
www.trotters.co.uk

'*Trotters* is renowned for being a 'one-stop-shop for children', providing high quality clothes, shoes (with a train for children to sit on while having shoes fitted, and then pretend to drive), books, toys, presents and even hairdressing – children have a lovely aquarium to gaze at as a distraction from the task in hand! The store is newly opened in Guildford following the successes of its three other London stores.'
Emma, mum of Charlotte and Louis

Shoes

Clarks Shoe Shop
108 High Street   *25-26 Friary Centre*
GU1 3HQ   *GU1 4YN*
(0844) 499 3135   *(0844) 499 9035*
www.clarks.co.uk

'Good range of reasonably priced, professionally fitted children's shoes. Staff are knowledgeable and friendly.'
Kris, mum of Olivia and Victoria

'I have bought all my daughter's shoes from *Clarks* so far as they have a good

Shopping

selection and are competitive on price. If you have young children and buggies I suggest that you go to the store in the *Friary* as the children's section in the store on the High Street is downstairs and there isn't a lift.'
Katherine, mum of Holly and Hazel

Russell & Bromley
84 High Street
GU1 3HE
(01483) 504879
www.russellandbromley.co.uk

'I always go to *Russell & Bromley* for my son's shoes as there is a wide stock range including *Clarks* and *StartRite*. The children's department is upstairs. However, there is an area under the stairs where buggies can be left and now that I have a running toddler, I am glad that he can be contained within the shop and cannot easily run out into the street. The store operates a ticket system, and staff are usually quick to serve you, even at the weekend when there seem to be lots more staff on duty. They check sizing thoroughly and always get a more senior and/or experienced member of staff to check the fitting. They are also happy to check current shoes, and they do tell you honestly if they think you have a few more weeks of growing space left or if it is time to buy new ones. The shoes can be a bit on the expensive side, but I feel that the service justifies this. You can get some real bargains in the sale.'
Lisa, mum of Thomas

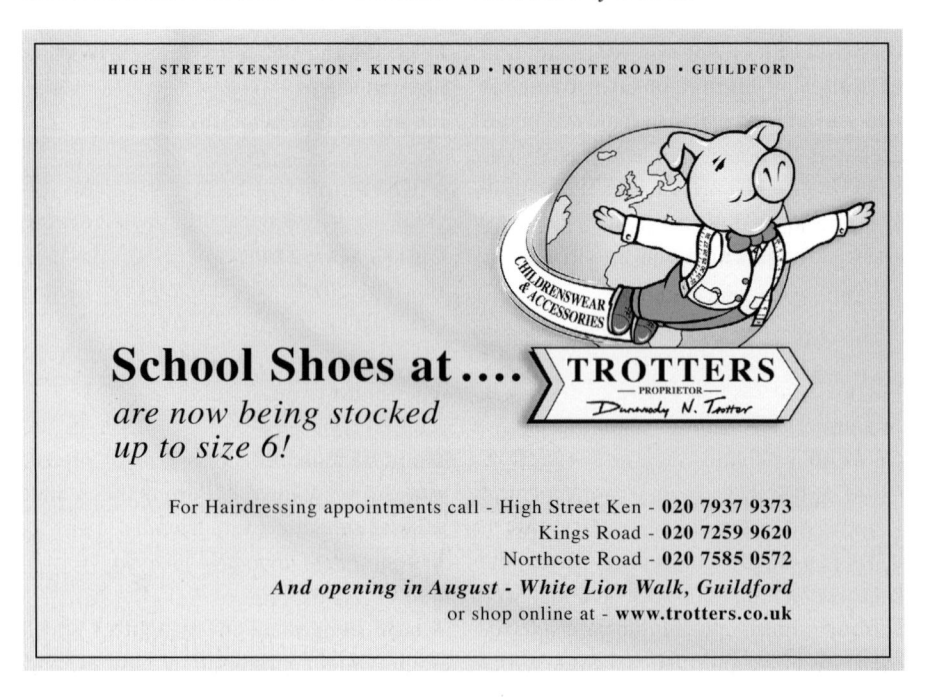

HIGH STREET KENSINGTON • KINGS ROAD • NORTHCOTE ROAD • GUILDFORD

School Shoes at....
are now being stocked up to size 6!

TROTTERS
— PROPRIETOR —
Dunnaody N. Trotter

For Hairdressing appointments call - High Street Ken - **020 7937 9373**
Kings Road - **020 7259 9620**
Northcote Road - **020 7585 0572**
And opening in August - White Lion Walk, Guildford
or shop online at - **www.trotters.co.uk**

Shopping

Trotters
Unit 6 White Lion Walk
GU1 3DN
01483 454668
www.trotters.co.uk

'*Trotters* stocks *StartRite* shoes, as well as ballet and football shoes, wellies and slippers. Professional fitters are on hand for correct sizing and fitting.'
Emma, mum of Charlotte and Louis

Baby Essentials and Maternity Wear

Boots
85-89 High Street
GU1 3DS
(01483) 572114/567928
www.boots.com

'*Boots* stocks an excellent range of feeding equipment and other 'baby kit', a small but nice range of baby clothes and a good selection of own brand and *Early Learning Centre* toys. The store even supplies free nappies in the baby changing room.

I have found that if you are shopping with a pushchair, it is easier to access the store down the ramp from the side entrance on Swan Lane. This is because the baby department, nappies, children's clothing, pharmacy and baby feeding/changing facilities, are all on the lower ground floor. '
Lisa, mum of Thomas

'The rear entrance has a ramp for easy pushchair use and there is a lift in the centre of the store. There are good baby changing facilities at lower ground floor level with complimentary nappies and wipes; there are also bottle warmers and an area for feeding.'
Vicki, mum of George and Finlay

'*Boots* does have a baby changing facility but be aware that there are no toilets. I did find this off-putting because normally when I need to change Jessica I could do with going to the toilet too!! The *Mini Mode* baby clothes range is great and reasonably priced too, although it is small.'
Linda, mum of Jessica

Blooming Marvellous
18 White Lion Walk   23 Oakdene Parade
GU1 3DW   Cobham
(0845) 458 7422   KT11 2LR
   (0845) 458 7428
www.bloomingmarvellous.co.uk

'This is a great shop for all sorts of things, although not cheap. I love its maternity clothes (nice and trendy) and I have also bought a few baby items such as feeding pillow, personalised items for family, babygros, baby journal book, etc., the list is endless! However, I would say that the store only stocks smaller sized nursing bras so ladies that are well endowed (like me, I am afraid!) would not be able to buy these here. Staff in the Guildford store are extremely helpful too. I would recommend getting the brochure sent to your home address because on a regular basis I seem to receive 10% off vouchers too, which are extremely useful and you can spend them

Shopping

either online or in store. There are no toilets or baby feeding facilities though.' (Guildford branch)
Linda, mum of Jessica

'Very friendly, helpful staff and some surprising bargains at their regular sales.' (Cobham branch)
Vicki, mum of George and Finlay

Formes
8 Tunsgate Square
GU1 3QZ
(01483) 454777
www.formes.com

'Beautiful French maternity apparel. The only downside is it's rather expensive. I found the way round this was to buy a couple of really fabulous pieces that will go with absolutely everything (black trousers and white lightweight jumper) and wear them constantly. I've now passed my trousers on and they're still going strong. They fitted well as I both increased and decreased in size after the birth and made me feel very smart.'
Sonya, mum of Eleanor and Charles

'*Formes* stocks gorgeous maternity clothes, which are fashionable, stylish, comfortable and well made. Unless you have pots of cash, I would say that their clothes are more for special occasions. I bought an outfit from there when I was 14 weeks pregnant and was getting just that little bit too big for 'normal' clothes, and I was still wearing it at 39½ weeks to Christmas parties. The trousers can be a bit on the long side though, and are probably better suited to women about 5'6" tall and above, unless you are handy with a sewing machine, or know someone who is.'
Lisa, mum of Thomas

JoJo Maman Bébé
The Friary Centre	*31 Oakdene Parade*
Level 2	*Cobham*
GU1 4YN	*KT11 2LR [NEW]*
(01483) 455390	*(01932) 865067*

www.jojomamanbebe.co.uk

'The shop sells baby essentials up to the age of five. If you sign up for *JoJo*'s e-mails you get offers most weeks for all your baby essentials, a lot of it with free postage and packing. The advantage of visiting the store is you can see the goods 'in the flesh' and if you've seen what you want in the catalogue, but it is not in store, the staff will order it in and you can pick it up in the store.'
Sonya, mum of Eleanor and Charles

'Too many gorgeous things. There are great sleepsuits with pop-over mits for scratchy babies with eczema. You can also buy through mail order.'
Lisa, mum of Lewis, Scarlett, Dylan, Saffron, Jude, and Reuben

'This shop stocks a selection of maternity wear, and some beautiful children's clothes and gifts, although it doesn't carry its whole catalogue range. The shop is ideal if you don't mind paying a little bit more than in other high street stores.'
Liz, mum of Elinor

Shopping

Mothercare – Guildford
12c North Street
GU1 4AF
(01483) 467240
www.mothercare.com

'*Mothercare* has a good clean changing room at the rear of the store. No toilet for toddlers, but three changing bays and a bench or armchair for breastfeeding mums.'
Sonya, mum of Eleanor and Charles

'Although the selection is smaller than the Weybridge branch I tended to use *Mothercare*'s feeding room a lot. It was clean and quiet. It had two baby changing mats, seating and bottle warmers. I found it very handy in the first few months when my confidence in breastfeeding in public was not great and I knew I could just nip in there.'
Lynn, mum of Ella

'There are probably lots of reviews of this shop, however I just wanted to add how impressed with their service we have been.

One particular instance was when my daughter was just born and had a snuffly nose and I wanted a nasal aspirator. *Mothercare* didn't have any in but the girl on the till told me exactly what I needed, as in my just post-birth state I couldn't remember what it was called, and assured me that I could get them in *Boots*. As it was, I'd just been to *Boots* and was met with blank looks but after speaking to the

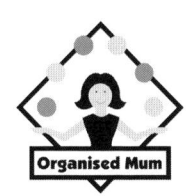

Brand new range of calendars and diaries now available from Organised Mum

Call 0845 644 7507 or visit
www.organised-mum.co.uk

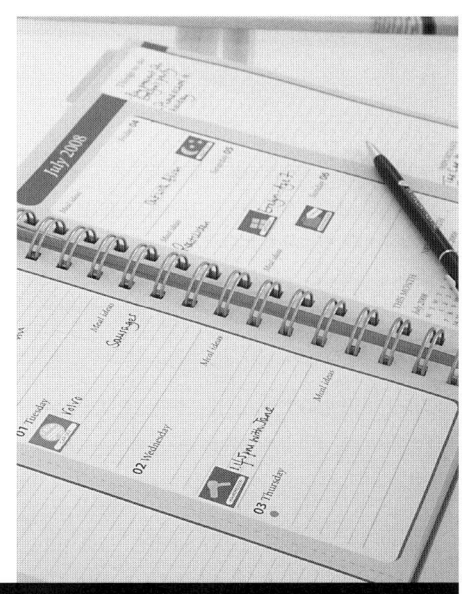

Calendars and diaries to organise your life

127

Shopping

lady at *Mothercare* I had the confidence to try again at *Boots* and this time managed to get one.'
Jacqui, mum of Harry and Megan

Mothercare World
*The Paddock Retail Park
Sopwith Way
Brooklands
Weybridge
KT13 0XR
(01932) 355069
www.mothercare.com*

'Brooklands is home to *M&S*, *Tesco* and *Mothercare World* [among other shops] and is ideal for a 'mooch' around. It is the largest *Mothercare* that I am aware of in the area, and when looking for prams the staff were very helpful and friendly. There is also a small in-house *Clark*s shoe shop. *Tesco* also has a coffee shop so you can combine a bit of retail therapy with that much needed coffee!' (Note: *Mothercare World* also houses a maternity wear section).
Lynn, mum of Ella

E. Moss Ltd. Traditional Pharmacy
*1 The Friary Centre
GU1 4YL
(01483) 579280
www.alliancepharmacy.co.uk*

'Useful for sourcing those remedies Granny swears by (*Bickiepegs*, teething granules etc.) It also dispenses normal prescriptions.'
Charlotte, mum of Noah

Toys and Books

Carousel
*1 Kings Road
Shalford
GU4 8LE
(01483) 893220
www.carouseltoyshop.co.uk*

'*Carousel* is small toy shop in Shalford, adjacent to the railway station and near to another toy shop (*Enchanted Wood*). It's usually easy to park right outside. The staff are really helpful and have stock stored nearby.
They have a good range of toys with some unusual items that can make interesting gifts.'
Rachel, mum of Amy, Thomas and Ella

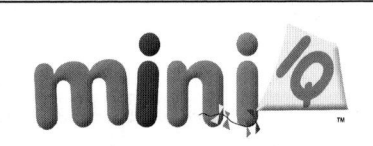

---

mini

Educational but FUN

Books, toys and games
for babies and children aged 0 - 12
To book your own coffee morning,
evening party or toddler group visit,
set up your own Party Plan business
by joining us, or to place an order,
please contact:
Sarah Clarke (01252) 851031
sarah.clarke@care4free.net

Shopping

The Disney Store
37-38 The Friary Centre
GU1 4YN
(01483) 440393
http://disneystore-shopping.disney.co.uk/

'This store is great for 'bribing' three-year-olds with a quick look round for behaving well while having feet measured at the *Clarks* opposite! It stocks all current *Disney* film merchandise but be warned you could find yourself leaving with all manner of colourful lunch bags, beach towels, toys or dressing up clothes!'
Jenny, mum of Imogen and Harrison

Early Learning Centre
14-15 North Street
GU1 4AF
(01483) 505138
www.elc.co.uk

'This is well used as a little pit stop on my way to library singing ('*Baby Bounce and Rhyme*' – see *Things to Do*). Ella loves running around usually with one of the toy buggies, or playing with whatever other toys are out for demonstration. The staff don't seem to mind children running around and enjoying themselves. You need to be vigilant if they are playing near the entrance, as the doors are nearly always open.'
Leena, mum of Ella

'The *ELC* is great for baby and preschool toys and has a fantastic painted ceiling to amuse babies in buggies! There are always lots of toys on display for children to play with, and there is a toilet and changing room at the rear right-hand side of the shop. *ELC*'s returns policy is excellent and will replace toys up to one year old if faulty no questions asked!'
Jenny, mum of Imogen and Harrison

Enchanted Wood
3-5 Kings Road   5 East Street
Shalford   Farnham
GU4 8JUGU9 7RX
(01483) 570088   (01252) 722222

10-12 Petworth Road
Haslemere
GU27 2HR
(01428) 648900
www.enchanted-wood.co.uk

'A large toy shop in Shalford, adjacent to the railway station and near to another toy shop (*Carousel*). Usually it's easy to park right outside. The shop has a good stock of *Lego*, *playmobil* and many other quality toys and helpful staff. My children find plenty to amuse themselves while I shop.' (Note: *Enchanted Wood* in Shalford is also home to the NCT library).
Rachel, mum of Amy, Thomas and Ella

The Entertainer
13b North Street
GU1 4AF
(0870) 9055130
www.theentertainer.com

'Often items are marked down dramatically – say, a *Barbie* figure from a less-recent *Barbie* film might be £3.00 instead of

Shopping

£20.00. If your children don't mind that it's not the newest, hippest, latest-out toy, it's worth a trawl through *The Entertainer* if you are passing, to see what deals are on.'
Kris, mum of Olivia and Victoria

Guildford Comics and Games
64b Chertsey Street
GU1 4HL
(01483) 304781

'Check out this small, independent store for lots of boxed games, jigsaws, board games and for the older 'children', role-playing games like *Dungeons and Dragons* (some of which are frequently being played in the back of the shop). Prices are competitive, e.g. it was the cheapest place I found to buy *Jenga*. Do not be put off by the tunnel-like entrance, pop in on your way past the pedestrian walkway to York Road car park; it's almost opposite Martyr Road.'
Sonya, mum of Eleanor and Charles

Toys'R'Us
The Peacocks Centre
Church Street West
Woking
GU21 6HD
(01483) 726449
www.toysrus.co.uk

'There are well-trained young staff in the *Babies'R'Us* section, who are all terribly helpful. Good value products and deals with a good cross section of the baby equipment market. It's a great one stop shop!'
Vicki, mum of George and Finlay

'I would describe *Toys'R'Us* as having the feel of a toy supermarket. There are very few toys that are set up for children to "road test" or play with in the store, but it has a huge range of most things. The store opens late in the evenings, which is handy for shopping trips without demanding children in tow, especially leading up to Christmas!'
Lisa, mum of Thomas

Waterstones
71-73 High Street   35-39 North Street
GU1 3DY   GU1 4TE
(01483) 536366   (01483) 302919
www.waterstones.co.uk

'This is one of our favourite places in Guildford and we always end up here for some rest and recuperation on any shopping trip. On the ground floor there is a large children's section with a rocking horse and a fish tank as a great distraction. There is a toilet with baby changing facilities on this floor as well. If you go to either the first or second floors there are some very comfortable sofas that are away from the main body of traffic in the shop and make a surprisingly peaceful and private place to feed young babies or just to sit and rest. There is also a café on the first floor if you are in need of refreshment.'
Katherine, mum of Holly and Hazel

'This is a favourite stop because of the fish tank in the children's section, and there are also toilets on the first floor which don't tend to have long queues.'
Sally, mum of James

ENCHANTED WOOD
CHILDREN'S STORES
SO MUCH MORE THAN A TOY STORE

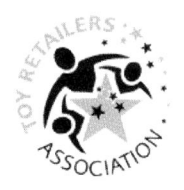

**Regional Winner
Toy Retailer of the Year Award
2005 and 2006**

Grobags   Leather Starter Shoes   Buggy Boards   New Baby Gifts
Fisher Price   Duplo   Orchard Toys   Plan Toys   Wooden Thomas
Tomy   Leapfrog   VTech   Dollhouses, Farms & Castles
Sylvanian Families   Baby Annabel   Galt   Hama Beads   Lego
Playmobil   Meccano   Hasbro   Mattel   Kettler Trikes & Go Karts
TP Activity Toys   Little Tikes   Guildford NCT Library (Shalford)
Party Bag Service

Call for our full colour catalogue

www.enchanted-wood.co.uk

FARNHAM	GUILDFORD	HASLEMERE
5 East Street	3-5 Kings Rd, Shalford	10-12 Petworth Road
01252 722222	01483 570088	01428 648900

Shopping

'The children's section often does '3 for 2' deals, and this is a great way to bulk-buy presents for all those children's parties!'
Kris, mum of Olivia and Victoria

WHSmith
56 High Street
GU1 3ES
(01483) 576217
www.whsmith.co.uk

Guildford Station
GU1 4UT
(01483) 568876

'There is a disabled toilet upstairs in WHSmith [High Street] where you can change babies.'
Tessa, mum of Daisy, Zach and Jake

Wooden It Be Lovely
22 Lion & Lamb Yard
Farnham
GU9 7LL
(01252) 716794
www.woodenitbelovely.net

'I just adore this toy shop; it is definitely our favourite. It sells only wooden toys that are beautifully handcrafted and CE tested. Wooden musical playthings, clocks, wooden dolls, rocking horses, ride-ons, scooters, hot air balloon lights, jigsaws and rattles – everything you could wish for.'
Nadine, mum of Noah and Luca

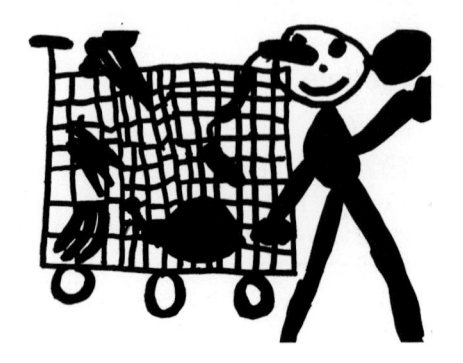

General Shops

Argos
193 High Street
GU1 3AW
(01483) 538666
www.argos.co.uk

13 North Street
GU1 4AF
(01483) 572121

'Huge store stocking pretty much anything you want. Good for lots of children's toys. Research online at home, reserve your goods at your nearest store and pop in to collect your order, thereby avoiding postage costs. Of course, the catalogue is in the store, but it's hard to ask a toddler to sit still while you navigate your way through the hundreds of pages. Prices not always the cheapest but you can always use your nectar points to pay for things.'
Sonya, mum of Eleanor and Charles

IKEA
Valley Park
Purley Way
Croydon
CR0 4UZ
(0845) 355 1144
www.ikea.co.uk

'This may seem like a strange choice, but I am something of an *IKEA* devotee, and although I prefer child-free evening trips to *IKEA* (Croydon is open until midnight), it's not a bad place to take the

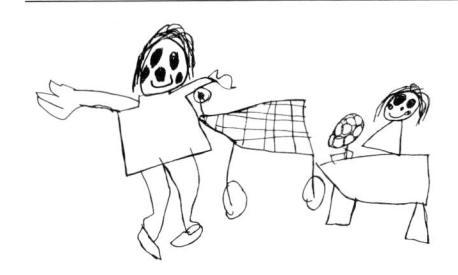

kids. Family parking spaces and large lifts make accessibility easy enough. The canteen caters well for feeding little people; there is a breastfeeding area, bottle warming facilities, and children's meals start from 75p. There is also a plentiful supply of highchairs, disposable bibs plus a children's play area. *IKEA* has a good range of children's products including toys, furniture, bedding, lighting and storage. I would highly recommend a visit (with or without the kids in tow) if you are planning to kit out a nursery on a budget.'
Louise, mum of James

The Friary Centre
GU1 4YT
(01483) 503773
http://guildford.org.uk/friarycentre

'As you would expect from a covered shopping centre *The Friary* is mostly buggy-friendly, except for *Topshop* where there are a lot of steps to navigate. The toilets at the rear of the ground floor have recently been spruced up, and there is now a cubicle with two toilets so you can go in with your child. There is even room for a small lightweight buggy too.'
Katherine, mum of Holly and Hazel

Woolworths
17-21 Friary Street
GU1 4EH
(01483) 452228
www.woolworths.co.uk

'Inexpensive children's clothing and lots of dressing up outfits. Upstairs (using the small lift) is the toy section. Competitively priced and all the popular toys of the moment stocked. No toilets. The nearest I've found are either in *Debenhams* or *The Friary Centre*.'
Sonya, mum of Eleanor and Charles

'Useful children's clothes section, some heavily 'logoed' but others more anonymous – nice, soft plain-coloured bodysuits, soft jackets for babies, pretty dresses. Good for cheap summer wear, dressing-up costumes and great for Wellington boots (starting in very small sizes for small, fast toddlers like mine). Also a big range of inexpensive toys and the kitchen department is good for plastic boxes etc. Tiny lift.'
Victoria, mum of Catherine.

Online/Catalogues

Abel & Cole
(08452) 626262
organics@abel-cole.co.uk
www.abel-cole.co.uk

'I have been a big fan of *Abel & Cole* for a few years now. They have never failed to provide first rate fresh organic produce to my door. The service is excellent, and the

Shopping

website is good. There is a guide to help you choose a suitable box for your needs and you can tell them your dislikes so they will substitute them with something else. There is a weaning box especially for those 'puree months'.
Liz, mum of Thomas

Aspace.co.uk
(0845) 872 2400
www.aspaceuk.com

'Top quality furniture. Expensive, but it does have sales and is perfect when you are looking for something special or distinctive for your little ones' rooms.'
Liz, mum of Thomas

Boden (mini)
(0845) 677 5000
www.boden.co.uk

'Good quality clothing for boys and girls. Slightly expensive, but nice to get some things that are a bit different. They have some very good sales.'
Liz, mum of Thomas

The Book People
(0845) 602 3030/4040
www.thebookpeople.co.uk

'*The Book People* is a fantastic mail order and internet company that offers great books at amazingly low prices. It is not a book club so you do not commit to anything. You simply buy books when you want them. The company sends out a monthly magazine but there is always loads more choice if you look on the internet. Books always arrive very quickly and there is usually a freepost offer if you order over a certain value of books – easily done if you get one or two friends to order with you. There is a good range of both children's and adults' books.'
Jo, mum of Thomas, George and Rebecca

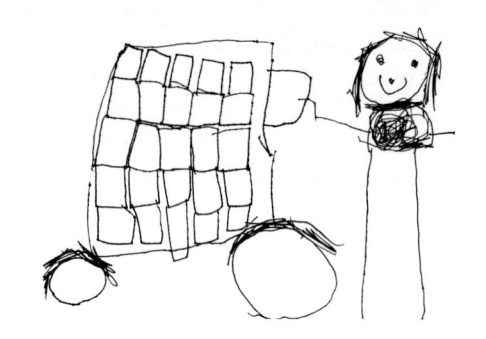

Bump to 3
(0844) 557 3007/2983
www.bumpto3.co.uk

'The makers of the *Grobag*®, those invaluable sleeping bags for little ones, provide an efficient service when it comes to delivering. They also sell other useful products such as wet weather garments, feeding products and sleeping accessories.'
Liz, mum of Thomas

Great Little Trading Company
(0870) 850 6000
enquiries@gltc.co.uk
www.gltc.co.uk

'A great catalogue company that delivers next day on most in stock products and

offers a wide range of nursery and toddler bedroom furniture and decorations, practical baby equipment and great garden toys – a bit pricey but lovely quality and design.'
Jenny, mum of Imogen and Harrison

Kiddicare
www.kiddicare.com

'An enormous range of equipment. Very, very keen prices, rarely beaten on the net and free delivery. *Kiddicare* also price matches. Delivery is very quick and the company holds a very large stock.'
Sonya, mum of Eleanor and Charles

Naturebotts
(0845) 226 2186
www.naturebotts.co.uk

'Lovely range of ecological/natural products from a small business. The company sells *Moltex Oko* [see Services – 'Eco-friendly disposables'] the unbleached, biodegradable nappies and the lovely smelling *Earth Friendly* baby skincare range plus a lot more. The nappies might not be quite as cheap as other main online competitors but you get good personal service and staff are very helpful if you ring them.'
Sonya, mum of Eleanor and Charles

'I bought *Moltex Oko* nappies for both my babies from *Naturebotts* [see Services – 'Eco-friendly disposables']. I was always very happy with the service. I always stocked up, so bought two boxes of nappies (three packets per box) as this kept the cost down a bit, and they always arrived the day after I ordered them (as long as I didn't order them just before a weekend). Whenever I left a message on the phone, the staff called me back very quickly, and they kept a record of my order, and how often I needed to order, which I found very helpful.

They were the only nappies that didn't irritate my children and I liked to feel I was doing a bit for the environment by using biodegradable nappies (although, I have to say, I didn't invest in a wormery for the purposes of biodegrading).'
Emma, mum of Charlotte and Louis

Ocado
(0845) 399 1122 / (0845) 656 1234
www.ocado.com

'Until William was a year old, I still loved going supermarket shopping, but when he started grabbing things and then on my return to work, I became a home shopping expert.

Having tried the others, Ocado is my absolute favourite, and because I am more disciplined in my shopping and keep to my list, I spend less and waste less. Orders over £75.00 have free delivery, and there are one hour delivery slots. You can make lists online, claim for refunds if you haven't been sent what you ordered (very rare!) and the website has recipes for when your sleep-deprived brain can't work out what you should be cooking/ordering/eating! I can now do my order in 10-15 minutes, and because the bags

Shopping

arrive colour coordinated, the green freezer bags get put away first, then the red fresh stuff, and any purple bags can wait until after bed/meal/nappy change.'
Claire, mum of William

Partybox
www.partybox.co.uk

'A good, wide range of party goods that you can order online and then if, like me, you've left it a bit late and want to be sure to have your goods in time for the party, you can drive over to Knaphill and pick everything up. Prices seemed to be similar to other websites but of course you save the £3.60 delivery charge if you go and collect yourself.'
Sonya, mum of Eleanor and Charles

Riverford
(01803) 762720
www.riverford.co.uk

'A lot of parents suddenly think more about organic food when their children get to weaning stage, and I was no different. Starting shopping with *Riverford*, which sources all organic and mostly British food, makes me feel better about the small range of fruit and vegetables that William will eat. The seasonal fruit and vegetables supplied in their boxes can be delivered weekly, fortnightly or monthly, and there are lots of extras that you can order on a regular or ad-hoc basis, like eggs, milk, extra fruit or veg, organic wine, chocolate and books.

After a couple of years of trying different combinations, I now have a mini box one week and a fruit and veg the alternate week. It's great to see William rooting through when it arrives to find what interesting things there are to eat.'
Claire, mum of William

Tickseed
(01780) 450790
david@tickseed.co.uk
www.tickseed.co.uk

'A lovely range of toys that aren't necessarily available on the high street and at good prices. Stock ranges from party bag/stocking fillers to musical instruments, soft toys, craft kits and science projects. A personal service from a small family business.'
Sonya, mum of Eleanor and Charles

---

* * * * * * * * * * * * * * * *

Baby Bargains of Ash

We buy and sell quality, as new, baby equipment

Toys - Clothes - Cots - Cribs - Prams - New Bedding - Strollers & Gates

Opening Times:
Tues-Thurs & Sat: 10.00am -4.00pm
Fri: 10.00am - 2.30pm
Mon & Sun: Closed

FREE OFF ROAD PARKING

Tel: 01252 326916
59 Guildford Road, Ash,
Aldershot, GU12 6BQ

* * * * * * * * * * * * * * * *

Shopping

Vertbaudet
(0844) 842 0000
www.vertbaudet.co.uk

'A good variety of clothes and furniture for children of all ages. All reasonably priced.'
Liz, mum of Thomas

Second Hand Bargains

NCT Nearly New Sales
St Joseph's Church Hall
York Road
GU1 4AX
(01483) 237778 / (08704) 609641
www.nctguildford.org.uk
[Note: sales are in the spring and autumn. See *All About the NCT*.]

'Great fun to help out and if you do, you get early pickings on the day. But even if you just attend to buy there are some great bargains; I have had some lovely clothes, shoes and kit for my two at a fraction of the retail cost.

Definitely worth a visit and definitely worth contributing a little of your time. It is a great way to meet new people.'
Vicki, mum of George and Finlay

'Always great for fantastic clothing, equipment and toy bargains! The sale is really well organised with all items grouped together. For example, clothes are separated onto different rails according to size, with girls' clothes on one side of the room and boys' on the other.'
Lisa, mum of Thomas

'I've bought whole summer wardrobes for £30.00, *Grobag*® sleeping bags for a third of the price of *Ebay*, and toys that look like they've only been sucked once or twice. Sharpen your elbows though; getting what you're looking for before someone else does is serious business.'
Rosie, mum of Lily

Farnborough Car Boot Sale
Pinehurst car park
Farnborough Road
GU14 7JZ
(01252) 398292 / (01252) 398398
mike.bamber@rushmoor.gov.uk
Sundays 11.00-16.00

'This is the best car boot sale I have ever been to for children's clothes and toys. I enjoy both buying and selling, especially if selling with a friend as you share the entrance fee of £8.00, so then you only need to sell a few items before you're in credit (if you don't spend it all again that is). On a rainy day you get just as many buyers as half of the sale is undercover. I always think that there are more girls' clothes there than boys' clothes but I have never returned home empty handed.'
Nadine, mum of Noah and Luca

Seasons Nearly New
2B The Square
Onslow Village
(01483) 504463

'This is a great little shop where you can both buy and sell children's toys and children's and women's clothing,

Shopping

including maternity wear and shoes. The clothing is always in good condition and very reasonably priced. The stock changes rapidly so it is worth popping in on a regular basis. There is a small table and chairs with paper and crayons to keep little ones amused while you browse and try things on.'
Katherine, mum of Holly and Hazel

Public Toilets and Changing Facilities

'Guildford Town Centre toilets include:

North Street
- *Early Learning Centre* – separate toilet and changing/feeding room at rear right-hand side of shop.
- *House of Fraser* – first floor next to children's department.
- Public toilets on corner of North Street and Ward Street, opposite library. (No toilets in the Library).

White Lion Walk
- *Next* – next to the tills in the women's department is a public toilet (from before *Next* was there). The only problem is the cubicles are too narrow for a pram/buggy.

Friary Centre
- Top floor near restaurants and bottom floor near the rear escalator.

High Street:
- *Debenhams* – ladies and disabled on ground floor at rear right-hand side by restaurant, and men's, ladies, disabled and baby changing facilities on homeware (second) floor.
- *M&S* – first floor near ladies underwear.
- *Waterstones* – ground floor at the rear right-hand side behind the children's department, also a changing room.
- *Tunsgate Café* in the *Tunsgate Centre*.

Upper High Street
- McDonald's.'

Helen, mum of Dominic and Laura

Civic Hall car park

'As far as public toilets go, the *Civic Hall* car park provides clean, well-maintained toilets that you can get into with a buggy, although you do have to leave it outside the cubical. I've never had to queue, either when pregnant or with toddlers in tow, which is great.'
Jenny, mum of Imogen and Harrison

Tunsgate

'Tunsgate [outside on the road] has a public toilet next to Heals. Not the cleanest, but it's convenient in that you don't have to go into a big store and wait for lifts.'
Sonya, mum of Eleanor and Charles

Friary Centre

'The ground floor toilets are great if you have children with you. There is an

automatic sliding door into the toilet area so you don't have to struggle with a pushchair. There is also a family toilet with a child-size toilet as well as an adult one, plus two sinks in it, one child height. Flushes and taps are all touch sensitive ones so easy for children to use.'
Louise, mum of Joseph and Emilia

'I have often ended up in the top floor toilets, usually when my little boy has been caught short, and because I've only just found out (working on this book!) that ground floor toilets in *The Friary* existed! I find the top floor ones easy to get to, as long as I don't have to wait too long for a lift, and even with a buggy they are easily navigable, although you can't take a buggy into the cubicle with you. There is a separate baby changing room/disabled toilet, but you have to ask restaurant staff or cleaner for a key.'
Emma, mum of Charlotte and Louis

Peacocks Centre, Woking

'These are very good with two toilets available. Great changing facilities.'
Lisa, mum of Lewis, Scarlett, Dylan, Saffron, Jude, and Reuben

Baby Changing

'I have been to *Boots*, *Mothercare* and *M&S*. *Mothercare* is the cleanest and newest out of these, has good seating for breastfeeding and feels large and spacious for nappy changing too. There is also a bottle-warming facility. However, it can feel rather clinical when you are sitting feeding. *Boots* offers free nappies (just newborn ones I think) but it doesn't seem to be cleaned as often as the *Mothercare* room and I have sometimes seen overflowing bins, which is not much fun when you are breastfeeding!'
Lucy, mum of Lily

6
Eating Out

Kelley Friel

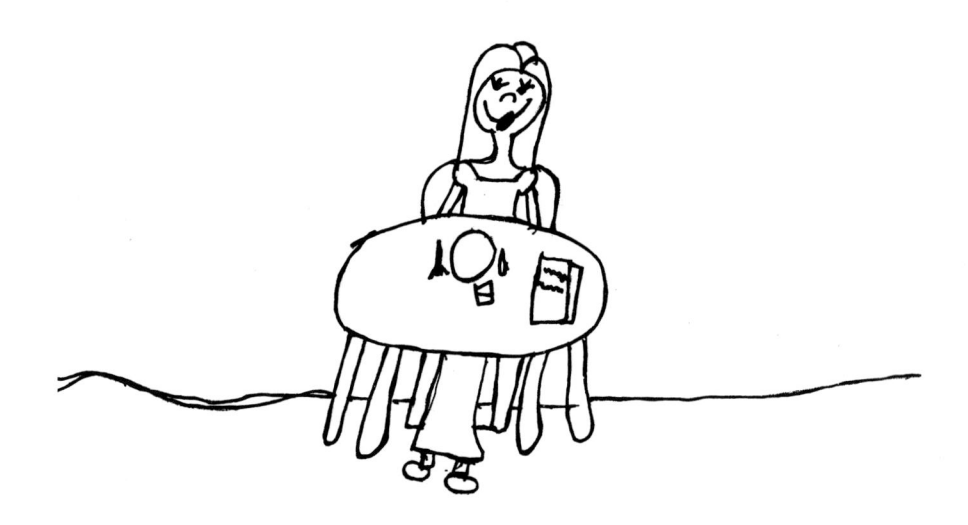

In the 18 months since our daughter was born, we have taken her to a number of different cafés and restaurants, and she's now quite fond of going out – and enjoys people-watching. I would recommend starting when the kids are young, both to get them accustomed, and for you and your partner to practise the precision operation needed to gather all the necessary toys, food and feeding equipment in addition to the normal changing gear.

You will likely find that your criteria for choosing a restaurant or café completely changes when you consider taking a baby or toddler. Perhaps you trade a romantic atmosphere and long, leisurely meals for a location with high chairs, reasonably quick service, an appealing children's menu and enough background noise to hide those occasional toddler outbursts. But it is still possible to enjoy a nice meal out!

We have included reviews of restaurants, cafés, and pubs that other parents have found to be child-friendly. I encourage you to use these reviews as a good excuse to venture out and try new places with your little ones!

Bon appétit!

Eating Out

Restaurants

Ask
16-19 Chapel Street
GU1 3UL
(01483) 577027
www.askrestaurants.com

'We went to Ask for lunch recently with two buggies that were easily accommodated. Staff provided crayons and paper for our toddler. Very family-friendly.'
Jo, mum of James and Daisy

'Staff at this pizza and pasta restaurant happily provided high chairs, moved tables, and accommodated us in every way, even letting us in a few minutes early. The music playing in the background entertained Audrey and drowned out any 'little' noises. There is also a very nice changing area in the disabled toilet.'
Kelley, mum of Audrey

'There is a good selection of dishes, predominantly Mediterranean at this restaurant at the bottom of the high street. High chairs and baby-changing facilities are available, and staff are happy to provide hot water to warm food.'
Heather, mum of Jessica

Auberge
274 High Street
GU1 3JL
(01483) 506202

'The bar space downstairs is the perfect place during the day for groups of mums to get together with small infants and have a little something that is a cut above a 'Debs' stale pastry. There are comfy sofas and chairs, room for pushchairs (and it's empty in daytime), and it makes you feel like a stylish, free, young woman again. Plus it is excellent for people-watching and the staff are cool about breastfeeding.'
Paige, mum of Miranda and Leo

Bar Centro
1c Sydenham Road
GU1 3RT
(01483) 302888
www.barcentro.co.uk

'Bar Centro is a café-style restaurant where children are very welcome and staff usually make a fuss over them. There are no specific children's facilities (other than high chairs) or a kid's menu, but the food is very good.'
Rachel, mum of Amy, Thomas and Ella

Bel and the Dragon
United Reformed Church
Bridge Street
Godalming
GU7 3DU
(01483) 527333
www.belandthedragon-godalming.co.uk

'This restaurant is in a lovely setting in a converted church, located in the centre of Godalming. It has great gourmet food, and is a good place for special occasions. There is no children's menu *per se*, but child portions are provided from the main menu. As a more sophisticated

setting, which is reflected in the price, it is probably better suited to young babies and older children than toddlers, but you are made welcome.'
Jo, mum of Oliver and Jake

Blubeckers Mill House
North Warnborough
Nr Hook
RG29 1ET
(01256) 702953
www.blubeckers.co.uk

'This *Blubeckers* is a family-friendly restaurant about a 40-minute drive from Guildford. It is a good place for Sunday lunch, but pre-booking is advised. With good and reasonably priced children's (and adult's) menus, complete with high chairs, which come with balloons and colouring pens, *Blubeckers* is very child-friendly. There is a small playroom downstairs, which is more appropriate for young children than babies as it can get boisterous! There is also an outdoor playground for older toddlers and young children, providing a setting where Mum or Dad can finish their lunch in peace!'
Jo, mum of Oliver and Jake

Blubeckers at Gomshall Mill
Station Road (on the A25)
Gomshall
GU5 9LB
(01483) 203060
www.blubeckers.co.uk

'This is a lovely family restaurant in an old mill along the river. There is a wide range of reasonably priced delicious food, catering both for those with straightforward tastes and for those looking for a little more spice! And the children's menu is more varied than just the usual pasta and tomato sauce. The super staff make you and your children feel really welcome, providing children with their own helium balloon and kids' packs containing colouring and entertainment kits. Food comes quickly and once children are finished they can go and peer through the glass at the water as it rushes over the mill wheel and under the building. Changing facilities are a pull-down table in the disabled toilet.'
Sonya, mum of Eleanor and Charles

'*Gomshall Mill* is renowned as a child-friendly pub/restaurant. The staff go out of their way to please the kids; children have a special menu, plus crayons, entertainment books and balloons. The menu choice is excellent and, unusually, meals are always presented with vegetables or salad. The restaurant also has a disused waterwheel on display (through glass), a play frame and attractive garden at the rear. There is a car park opposite. Bookings are necessary.'
Debra, mum of Ben and Eddie

Café Rouge
8 Chapel Street
GU1 4AS
(01483) 451221
www.caferouge.co.uk

'A colouring activity page and crayons are provided for the kids, which makes

it worth a go as the kids have something to keep them amused. There is a good children's menu and high chairs are available. There is not much room for prams; you are expected to fold them up and leave them by the door. Toilets are up a few flights of stairs, but there are no changing facilities.'
Helen, mum of Dominic and Laura

Carluccio's Caffé
57-59 High Street
Esher
KT10 9RQ
(01372) 467459
www.carluccios.com

'The owners of this restaurant have clearly given thought to looking after little ones. The children's menu is well thought out and offers decent food instead of the usual rubbish some restaurants think you'll be happy to give your children. The chicken escalope with rosemary potatoes was very tasty.

If you order from the children's menu staff will bring a cup of breadsticks over immediately (hallelujah!) and children are also given coloured pencils and paper to entertain them. Great 'babyccinos' (milk froth with a little chocolate sprinkled on top) and of course fab food and drink for the adults. There is also a tempting range of their food on sale to take away.

There is also a branch in Kingston upon Thames – I only wish they would hurry up and open a branch in Guildford!'
Jacqui, mum of Harry and Megan

Brasserie Chez Gérard
260-262 High Street
GU1 3GL
(01483) 569199
www.brasseriechezgerard.co.uk

'One evening, when my husband was away and my eldest daughter was at a sleepover, Victoria (four and a half) and I decided to have an elegant ladies' evening out at *Chez Gérard*. Despite appearing terribly grown-up from the outside, inside the staff made quite an effort to be child-friendly. There was a straightforward children's menu, from which Victoria ordered a small-but-perfectly-formed battered 'Cod and Frites', and there was a very good activity pack to keep her busy while she waited. I was really pleased with my Salad Niçoise, which was very fresh and beautifully presented, and our waiter was pleasant and friendly.

High chairs are available but there isn't enough room to keep your buggy by your table, so you have to fold it up and put it out of the way. Our waiter held open the door for us upon our departure, so I didn't have to wrestle the buggy through on my own – a thoughtful touch which I always appreciate.

If you and your husband/partner ever get out on your own, it's also worth knowing that *Chez Gérard* has a real cocktail bar, with a real cocktail menu. It's a great destination for, say, post-cinema when you don't wish to go straight home.'
Kris, mum of Olivia and Victoria

Eating Out

Da Gennaro Italian Restaurant
94 Woodbridge Road
GU1 4PY
(01483) 452253
www.dagennaro.co.uk

'*Da Gennaro* is tucked away on the one way system that runs from the bottom of North Street past the old cinema. It looks totally inauspicious from the outside, but it is a wonderful place to enjoy great, freshly cooked Italian food with the kids. The owners are always welcoming and genuinely seem to enjoy having child visitors. We've eaten there at both lunch-time and early evening with our pre-schooler and new baby. They have a few high chairs, a big toilet with room to change (although no specific facilities) and they are always willing to do a child-sized portion.'
Julie, mum of Ben and Katie

Debenhams Restaurant / Café
64 Millbrook
GU1 3UU
(01483) 467532

'*Debenhams Restaurant* is exceptionally baby-friendly. There is plenty of space for prams (even if, like me, you are extremely uncoordinated with anything wheeled!) and there are two sizes of high chair so even babies unable to sit up can come out of their prams if necessary. There is a microwave for heating food/bottles and nobody complains if you settle yourself and pram before going up to get food/drink. There are jars of baby food available to buy, and the food ranges from sandwiches to hot meals. There are some toys in the corner and a view of the river from the windows or from the outside terrace. There are toilets next to the restaurant, but they are not wide enough for a pram.

The café in *Debenhams* is also on the ground floor. It is much smaller but there are high chairs (one of each size).

Debenhams has excellent baby-changing facilities on the second floor (including a bar in front of the changing mat, paper towels and sink – no toilets within the changing room, but they are right next door). There is a sign telling you to ask for staff assistance if you have a double buggy. The feeding room is attached to the changing room and consequently not fabulous, but I've not encountered any problems feeding in either the restaurant or the café.

If you have a *Debenhams* Gold Card you get 10% off any purchases in the café or restaurant.'
Katy, mum of Edward

'This is the only restaurant I've found in Guildford that has baby food and bottle-warming facilities along with other accessories like bibs and wipes etc., which makes it an excellent choice for babies and toddlers. It is in a great location, next to the river, so after eating you can go and feed the ducks or take a stroll.'
Pippa, mum of Max and Evie

'Just the best place in Guildford to go with tiny tots for lunch. There is a great range

of disposable food pots, bibs etc., and a microwave to heat your own food; or you can share your baked potato and beans. We had our first spontaneous meal out with the twins here (I only had beakers with me) it was a great experience and I enjoyed the sit down. Access for the double buggy was not bad and we felt welcome.'
Sue, mum of Chris, Dan, Matt and Pip

Giraffe
215-217 High Street
GU1 3BH
(01483) 300237
www.giraffe.net

'This was a lovely place to take the children. The food was lovely and freshly prepared, and there were some different and healthier choices than you would expect normally, although no set menu. Sophie loved her salmon and broccoli! The grown-up food was equally satisfying. The staff were very friendly and welcoming although it was very busy and felt a bit chaotic. High chairs were available, but surprisingly I couldn't find any changing facilities.'
Louise, mum of Sophie and Phoebe

'My husband and I ate at the Clapham location of this chain restaurant pre-baby and felt out of place without children. It is very child-friendly and reminiscent of the *Rainforest Café*. This will hopefully be a local solution for taking the family entourage out for a bite without worrying about bothering the other customers!'
Cathi, mum of Ben and Ella

Jo Shmo's
244-246 High Street
GU1 3JF
(01483) 535255
www.joshmos.com

'We have lately started going to *Joe Shmo's* regularly at the weekends, and there are always lots of families with young children. The food, which more or less accurately bills itself as 'American', is fresh, imaginative, well cooked, and in generous portions.

The children's menu, while not extensive, has better quality versions of the usual standbys: for example, the chicken strips are excellent breaded chicken 'nuggets' which even an adult would be happy to eat. The main menu features burgers, wraps, salads and more, and the raised dining area at the back is bright, airy and cosy. Staff are friendly and helpful.'
Kris, mum of Olivia and Victoria

Loch Fyne
Centenary Hall
Chapel St
GU1 3UH
(01483) 230550
guildford@lochfyne.net
www.lochfyne.com
[Special offers can be found on the website, where you can download vouchers or check which newspaper you need to collect vouchers from.]

'Behind the unimposing entrance to this excellent fish restaurant is an impressive interior to this renovated listed building. For seafood lovers, oysters and mussels are among the offerings, together with a good variety of fresh and smoked fish, much of it flown in from Scotland each morning. There is also a smaller selection of non-fish dishes.

High chairs are provided, and a generally relaxed and friendly atmosphere makes this a child-friendly venue. There are stairs up to the restaurant but a wheelchair lift is available. Baby-changing facilities are also provided. The restaurant is a short walk from Sydenham Road car park.'
Louise, mum of James

'This is a great place to eat and children are provided with colouring paper and crayons. Access is awkward as the main restaurant is located on the first floor, but staff are always available to help carry pushchairs [and there is a small lift]. There is a children's menu and a special lunch-time menu for adults for £10.00 [2007] which includes a starter and main course [see website].'
Becki, mum of Jack

Olivo Ristorante

53 Quarry Street
GU1 3UA
(01483) 303535

'This is a great grown-up restaurant where children are very welcome. There are no specific child facilities or menu, but my kids loved the pasta and pizza.'
Rachel, mum of Amy, Thomas and Ella

Pizza Express – Guildford

237-241 High Street
GU1 3BJ
(01483) 300122
www.pizzaexpress.co.uk

'Crammed with young families, *Pizza Express* wrote the book on family friendliness. Firstly, it is open for dinner during the crucial hours from 4.00 to 6.00 pm. Secondly, thoughtfully designed and executed children's activity packs are provided, which even my eight-and-a-half-year-old still looks forward to. Thirdly, there is a new [2007] dedicated children's menu that represents excellent value for money. Fourthly, the food is fresh, imaginative, high-quality, and equally appealing to adults. Fifthly, staff are friendly and welcoming. One drawback: it's impossible for smaller children to reach the sinks in the toilets for hand washing. Bring wipes!'
Kris, mum of Olivia and Victoria

'*Pizza Express* is very child-friendly – we often head there after 'Baby Bounce and Rhyme' at the library [see p46] so there are a few of us. Although the doors are open, the staff haven't always started serving food, but they are happy to let us settle in and serve us coffee while we peruse the menu.'
Sarah, mum of Benedict and Jolyon

'*Pizza Express* has always been a great family venue. Go there at tea time and you will see the restaurant gradually fill up with families with young children.

There is a fantastic children's 'Piccolo' menu, which allows the children to enjoy a proper three-course meal alongside the rest of the family: dough balls for starters, a choice of pizza or pasta, and ice cream desserts in edible baskets, and, to top it off, chocolate-dusted frothed milk in an espresso cup alongside your coffee course, all very good value.

In between, the kids are kept entertained with the free 'Piccolo pack' – a box with a threading card and shoelace, press-out-and-build animal, puzzles, colouring and crayons inside. There are high chairs for babies and toddlers, booster seats for preschoolers, a baby-changing room and, most important of all, sympathetic and on-the-ball servers who seem to love entertaining babies.

In the summer you can sit out in the conservatory or on the small patio. Our boys also love their revolving door, though there is a large door and ramp for pram access. The last time we went, we stayed for two hours with our two and four year old boys, and they were happy the whole time!'
Julie, mum of Eliot and Oliver

Pizza Express – Haslemere

1 Causeway Side
High Street
Haslemere
GU27 2JZ
(01428) 642245
www.pizzaexpress.co.uk

'*Pizza Express* on Haslemere's High Street is very child-friendly, with about six high chairs available and a baby-changing unit in the disabled toilet. The staff are always friendly and welcoming, paying just the right kind of attention to our children, and it is very popular with families.'
Kerry, mum of Joe and Lyla

Pizza Hut

12 North Street   *27 Woodbridge Road*
GU1 4AF   *GU1 1DY*
(01483) 300501   *(01483) 546454*
www.pizzahut.co.uk
[Review for North Street Restaurant. Woodbridge Road is collection/delivery.]

'*Pizza Hut* is fabulous for hassle-free dining with little ones. The staff are so used to families, they didn't bat an eye when my daughter spilled an entire glass of soft drink all over the table, seat and floor. They have colouring packs for the kids, the food is colourful, quick and filling, and it's easy to get in and out.'
Paige, mum of Miranda and Leo

Rajdoot Tandoori Restaurant

220 London Road
Burpham Parade
GU4 7JS
(01483) 451278
info@rajdoottandoori.com
www.rajdoottandoori.com

'This is one for younger children. Staff are friendly and more than happy to accommodate a sleeping tot in a pram. It is an excellent place to start venturing out in the evening with a small one in tow.'
Charlotte, mum of Noah

Eating Out

Strada
222 High Street
GU1 3JD
(01483) 454455
www.strada.co.uk
[Restaurant undergoing refurbishment at time of publication.]

'We adore *Strada*! Although it's not specifically family-oriented, and there's no children's menu, the atmosphere is special. The staff are so welcoming and friendly, and they will do a child's portion of anything on the menu. My two girls always order Penne con Bufala, and then proceed to studiously remove every trace of a vegetable from the sauce. There is something cosy and gentle about *Strada*, and the food is delicious!'
Kris, mum of Olivia and Victoria

'*Strada*'s friendly staff are very accommodating towards young children, and there always seem to be enough high chairs. There is currently a pull-down changing table in the female toilets.'
Leena, mum of Ella

TGI Friday's
2 North Street
GU1 4AA
(01483) 300133
1647@crww.com
www.tgifridays.co.uk

'*Friday's* does good food, but it can take forever to arrive. The service can be erratic even when the restaurant is empty. But high chairs can be provided, and there is enough space to cope with pushchairs. There are also kids' activity packs and balloons, and on a good day staff even do balloon-modelling for children.'
Jo, mum of Matthew

Wagamama
25-29 High Street
GU1 3DY
(01483) 457779
www.wagamama.com
[The website has a 'Noodle Doodlers' page for kids to have fun!]

'*Wagamama* has a really inventive children's menu, so if your child is terrified by anything unfamiliar, it may not work. Having said that, my very finicky eight-year-old really enjoyed the Chicken Katsu, which is strips of chicken in a crispy batter. It was served with sticky rice and shredded cucumber – so it looked very different from her usual fare, but she gamely picked up her kiddy chopsticks and devoured most of it. Also, it's such a noisy place that no one will notice the whinging, complaining, and howling coming from your end of the communal dining table!'
Kris, mum of Olivia and Victoria

'It's a great place to eat – there are large dishes, so it is excellent value for money. There is a children's menu, or you can ask for a second dish so you can share. There are plenty of high chairs and just about enough space for pushchairs, but get there early to avoid the lunch-time rush. The staff are friendly and can cope

with mess. Children's activity sheets and crayons are provided. The only downside is that there are no baby facilities and the toilets are upstairs.'
Jo, mum of Matthew

'*Wagamama* is very baby-friendly, and it is always bustling and a bit noisy, so if your little one is in a 'banging' or 'shouty' mood no one will really notice over the general hubbub. At very busy times you might have to wait a bit, but not long and the friendly staff will fit you on the end of a table where you can put one of their high chairs in easily. There is a junior menu, which is good value, and our little one loves the chicken with noodles – and the staff don't bat an eyelid when the noodles invariably end up on the floor (tip: noodles are more easily controlled than rice!)'
Tim, dad of Lily

Zizzi
274 High Street
GU1 3JL
(01483) 534747
www.zizzi.co.uk

'The staff are very friendly and high chairs are available. I've eaten there with both a pram (you need to ask the staff to let you in and out of the back entrance in the alley next to *Auberge* so you don't have to lug the pram up a flight of stairs) and with Edward in a car seat. Both times the staff were very helpful and both times they were quite happy for me to breastfeed. If you are breastfeeding, the banquettes along the walls are more comfortable than the central tables. The food is pretty standard Italian fare but easy to eat with one hand (the staff even cut up my pizza for me!!).'
Katy, mum of Edward

'This is a regular one for my husband and me with our two-year-old for an 'early-bird' meal at tea time. You can't book at the weekend, so tables are allocated on a first-come, first-served basis. It is usually full of families at this time, with lots of children. The high ceilings absorb any noise from the children; it is hardly noticeable. The food is good and reasonably priced: pizza, pasta, salads and lovely desserts. The staff are friendly and attentive and there are plenty of high chairs. There is no separate children's menu, but staff are happy to provide extra crockery and cutlery (or you can take your own) so that you can share your food with your little one(s). The kitchen and wood-fired oven is on show, which provides good entertainment and is a great distraction for a hungry toddler. The odd flambé-type event goes down a treat with our son who likes to watch the chefs in action!'
Lisa, mum of Thomas

'For almost a year, *Zizzi's* was our Tuesday lunch-time venue for our antenatal group. Entrance with buggies is through the car park of the building next door, but the staff were always very helpful – parking four to eight buggies, and providing us with high chairs and bottle-heating facilities. The sofas at the far end were great for discreet

feeding, and there is a disabled toilet with baby-changing on the ground floor. The food is great, with pizza and pasta in interesting variations, and salads for the summer months.'
Claire, mum of William

Cafés

Caffè Nero
House of Fraser (First Floor)
105-111 High Street
GU1 3DP
(01483) 511192
www.caffenero.com
[Alternative Caffè Nero venues – 69 High Street, GU1 3DY, (01483) 578811; 91 High Street, Godalming, GU7 1AW, (01483) 420826]

'*Caffè Nero* is very baby-friendly and there is plenty of space for prams. It is very unusual to go there and not bump into at least one other mum. The staff are friendly and are happy to warm food or bottles. There are also no bars to breastfeeding (I find the sofas and easy chairs very comfortable), and there are jugs of water/plastic cups that you can help yourself to. People frequently come and chat to you even if they don't know you and it is a good place to meet other mums and mums-to-be. The hot chocolate is tasty too!

The toilets are right next to the café and there are baby-changing facilities in the disabled toilet (there is often a queue). The paninis and sweet snacks are good. The one downside is that you can end up spending far more than you intended to

if you go out past the children's clothing section...!'
Katy, mum of Edward

'This has been one of my favourite places in town to take my son to since he was a baby. On offer is a good selection of delicious coffees, tasty sandwiches, salads and other healthy options, soft drinks and of course cakes, muffins and cookies. I find the staff very pleasant and helpful. *Caffè Nero* is located next to the lift and close to the changing room and toilet (always clean), which is very handy with the little ones. High chairs are also provided.'
Martina, mum of Oscar

'The coffee shop is next to a good changing room and disabled toilet complete with piped music. No problem with breast-feeding and right next to the baby clothes if you want some retail therapy.'
Sam, mum of Freya

'This is a real 'yummy mummy' haunt. On offer are lovely light bites, coffees and cakes. Drinking water is freely available, and staff are friendly and don't bat an eyelid at breastfeeding. Changing facilities are close by.'
Charlotte, mum of Noah

Café Net
2-3 Phoenix Court
GU1 3EG
(01483) 572041

'This is a hidden gem – central location, a great variety of decent food and drink

(though not the very cheapest), a large space, and comfy sofas for plunking toddlers onto. The only drawback is that there are no high chairs, but that hasn't stopped us coming frequently. It is also breastfeeding-friendly.'
Paige, mum of Miranda and Leo

'*Café Net* is great for taking a buggy (lots of space, big meals to share with kids) but there are no changing facilities and toilet cubicles are so small, pregnant women are liable to get trapped in them!'
Charlotte, mum of Noah

Café Revive
Marks & Spencer (First Floor)
61-65 High St
GU1 3EB
(01483) 502420

'This café always seems to have plenty of high chairs and space for pushchairs. The menu, while not huge, seems to have more selection and lower prices than coffee shops on the high street. Also on offer are kids' meals, and there is a baby-changing room on the same floor.'
Kelley, mum of Audrey

'There are delicious banana milkshakes at *Café Revive*!! It can get a bit busy but there are easy chairs at the back and the tables and chairs move easily if you need to weave a pram through. There are also high chairs. It is often full of mums and grandmas! There are changing facilities on the same floor and no one has complained about breastfeeding. The staff were very helpful recently when the lift broke, and they escorted any pram-pushers down in the stock lift.'
Katy, mum of Edward

'Living close to the town centre when my toddler was a baby, I used to frequent *Café Revive* because the staff were always so friendly and helpful. Pushing a buggy with a screaming baby desperate for food, the staff anticipate your needs, have a flask of water ready for the bottle and carry it over to your table for you, with an enormous hot chocolate with whipped cream! Just sooo helpful when it is impossible to carry a tray, get out your purse and push a buggy at the same time! Well done *M&S*!'
Jane, mum of Jessica

'*Café Revive* is excellent for light bites or a rest stop; the staff are helpful, there are plenty of high chairs, and it is fine to breastfeed if you don't mind an older audience. There are spacious baby-changing facilities (though a short way away), and the ladies' cubicles are big enough to get a buggy into.'
Charlotte, mum of Noah

'This has to be one of the best places to go with small children. It is a huge space with well-spaced tables, so there is no struggling to push the buggy in between, and it is rarely full, even on a weekend. For toddlers and older children, there is an excellent range of suitable food from great sandwich boxes to pasta and pizzas, which can be reheated for you. The staff

are always really helpful and friendly, and usually bring your tray over, particularly if you are a lone parent. There are lots of high chairs available, it is always clean, and the toilets/changing facilities are on the same floor. It is highly recommended – the only drawback is it's a bit pricey.'
Jude, mum of Maia

Café Zest
House of Fraser (top floor)
105-111 High Street
GU1 3DU
(01483) 534599

'*House of Fraser* is not the easiest of stores to navigate, due to mezzanine landings and poorly sited lifts. However, do go to the top floor for a special treat at *Café Zest*. It's not great for crowds of mums but perfect for a light lunch-time bite with a couple of friends. If you are lucky, you can get a terrace table – glorious on a sunny day. High chairs are available and staff are attentive and friendly.'
Vicki, mum of George and Finlay

Continental Café
6b Tunsgate Square
GU1 3QZ
(01483) 303619

'This café, located in the central courtyard of *Tunsgate* shopping centre, is an excellent meeting and lunch spot. There are plenty of tables, lots of high chairs and it is a self-service café with lots of reasonably priced choices. The only downside is that there isn't a baby-change facility, but a buggy always works!'
Colleen, mum of Freya

'This is a big space and very popular with parents, so nobody will mind much when you take up space with your buggy. The one drawback is that you have to go into the rather cramped café to get served, and it can be tricky to get back out with a tray and a buggy if you are on your own – a better choice if there are two or more of you as you can take turns. It's a long time since I had to heat milk or baby food, but I remember this being one of the few places where they don't mind microwaving for you. It is a pleasant, airy space for a longer break, and the food is relatively well priced. The big drawback is there are no changing facilities at all in *Tunsgate*, and the café toilet is tiny. If you need to do a change you have to go out of *Tunsgate* by *Heal's* and turn left to go to the public toilets (not awful but not my first choice)!'
Jude, mum of Maia

'This café gives you the feeling of being outside yet protected from the elements.

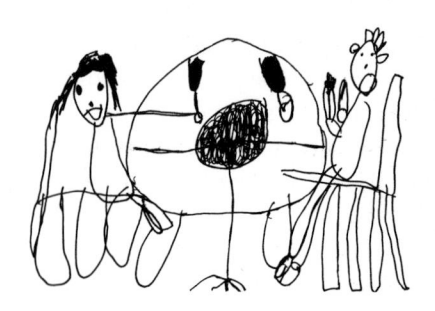

It is a good place to meet up for a drink and a bite to eat; you can move tables and chairs to fit the size of your group.'
Leena, mum of Ella

Costa Coffee
Waterstone's (1st Floor)
71-73 High Street *15-17 Swan Lane*
GU1 3DY *GU1 4EQ*
(01483) 578393 *(01483) 449545*
www.costa.co.uk
[Alternative Costa venues – The Spectrum Leisure Centre, GU1 1UP (01483) 443322; 11-14 Bridge Street, Godalming, GU7 1HY, (01483) 527430]

[Swan Lane review:]
'I have always found this a great place to head to for a spot of relaxed breastfeeding. It may be because of the way the tables are laid out and the subdued lighting, but I never feel too much on show, unlike other places which can be a little daunting. It has also proved to be a winner when you have a noisy fidgety toddler in tow, as they sell 'babyccinos' with marshmallows to bribe them to behave whilst you get on with feeding the baby. The staff are always very helpful. The changing room downstairs has been closed for over a year, but Boots is opposite and it has a good one.'
Jacqui, Mum of Harry and Megan

[*Waterstone's* reviews:]
'It is easy to get to by lift and ramp. It is not very big, but the pram was fine and breastfeeding is ok (although I do feel a little bit exposed and tend to use a shawl).'
Katy, mum of Edward

'*Costa Coffee* is great for people-watching if you manage to get one of the squidgy chairs by the window. It is a really nice relaxed environment with plenty of high chairs and staff are warm towards children – even offering 'babyccinos' (frothy milk – no caffeine!) Disabled toilets with baby-change facilities are on the ground floor.'
Vicki, mum of George and Finlay

'The staff are helpful and there are no problems with breastfeeding. Changing facilities are downstairs behind the children's book section, where the staff are very good at picking appropriate books for 12-month-olds!'
Sam, mum of Freya

Electric Theatre Café Bar
Onslow Street
GU1 4SZ
(01483) 444786
www.electrictheatre.co.uk

'This is a really good place for lunch away from the crowds. The food is great, and the bar is open at lunch-times. Breastfeeding felt ok here, and good changing facilities.'
Heather, mum of Jessica

Friary Shopping Centre Food Court and Boulevard Café
North Street
GU1 4YT
(01483) 503773 (Friary Centre)
www.guildford.org.uk/friarycentre

'The *Boulevard Café*, downstairs in the *Friary Centre*, has standard 'mall food'

153

Eating Out

(sandwiches, salads, jacket potatoes, pastries and cakes etc.) The staff are pretty friendly and happy to rearrange tables to allow you to fit prams in. There were no problems with breastfeeding, although I do take a shawl as you can feel a bit exposed.

There are good changing facilities at the bottom of the *Friary Centre*, as well as a feeding room. Personally, I prefer to feed in a coffee shop rather than a feeding room (partly because Edward tends to latch on for a good half hour each time!) but I know people who have spoken highly of the Friary one.

Upstairs (accessible by lift) there are a number of concessions in the *Food Court*, including burgers, jacket potatoes, Chinese food, pizza, smoothies, coffee, etc. There is plenty of seating, although some of it is up a step. There are more toilets and changing facilities right next to the *Food Court*.'
Katy, mum of Edward

'On the top floor of the *Friary Centre* there is an excellent *Food Court* where it is good to meet for lunch. There is a wide selection to choose from and for those just getting used to solids, the jacket potato stall means you can share a meal with your baby/toddler.

It is very child-friendly with plenty of high chairs and adequate changing facilities. There are also microwave facilities for those who prefer to bring their own food. It is an excellent idea for large groups.'
Sarah, mum of Benedict and Jolyon

Fruiti Boost Smoothie Bar
1 Chapel Street
GU1 3UH
(01483) 539595
www.fruitiboost.com

'My four-year-old asks for a smoothie when we are in town. This is our favourite one and very handy when walking to the castle grounds from the High Street. The staff are very friendly and can make a children's size smoothie with as many or as few fruits as you and your child would like. As well as smoothies, *Fruiti Boost* also sells freshly made juices, milkshakes and soups in winter. The ingredients are organic, and tired mums can have energy and vitamin boosts added to their drinks. I enjoy flicking through the gossip magazines while waiting for my drink to be made up.'
Thora, mum of Freyja

Garden Room
Castle Car Park
Sydenham Road
GU1 3RT
(01483) 577696

'We love this café – there is a massive selection of teas and coffees, really good cakes and pastries, smoothies etc. There is an imposed limit of two buggies in there at any time because of space restrictions, but it's a really nice place to meet up for a coffee if there aren't too many of you. There are a couple of high chairs but no changing facilities.'
Jo, mum of James and Daisy

Eating Out

Guildford Institute Restaurant
Ward Street
GU1 4LH
(01483) 562142
guildford-institute@surrey.ac.uk
www.guildford-institute.org.uk

'My daughter and I love eating here. The food is incredibly healthy (Guildford's only vegetarian restaurant – '*Beano's*') and very reasonably priced. The buffet lunch is served from 12.00 – 2.00 pm. The puddings are to die for! Unfortunately there is no lift and one has to negotiate a flight of stairs with a buggy, but it is well worth it once you reach the top. There is one high chair and it is possible to book it and seating in advance.'
Thora, mum of Freyja

Nell's Country Kitchen (Lucky Duck)
Middle Street
Shere
(01483) 202445

'This child-friendly café in the centre of gorgeous Shere has plenty of high chairs and a reasonably priced menu. When we went, there were several families with young children, and enough background noise and space between tables that we weren't too nervous that we were being too loud. There is a standard children's menu with jacket potatoes, beans on toast, etc. There is a space outside to leave prams, and a changing mat is provided that could just about work on the floor of the ladies' cubicle, but no changing table. The Shere public toilets are a short walk away with changing facilities.'
Kelley, mum of Audrey

'This is a family-run café/tea shop for a family lunch out. The quiche is delicious and comes with a huge plate of salad. They make their own delicious cakes and sell preserves and eggs. They also make meals for the freezer like lasagne or cottage pie. Once you've eaten, you can buy a bag of bread chunks and pop round the corner and feed the ducks in the stream (which is shallow enough for toddlers to wade in). Changing facilities are limited – when I went it was a changing mat on the floor in a tiny area.'
Sonya, mum of Eleanor and Charles

Riverbank Café Bar
Yvonne Arnaud Theatre
Millbrook
GU1 3UX
(01483) 569334
catering@yvonne-arnaud.co.uk
www.yvonne-arnaud.co.uk/eat.asp
[Note: there is also an à-la-carte restaurant at this venue]

'This is a spacious café with plenty of room for buggies. The food and snacks are nice, and there are high chairs and changing facilities in the ladies' toilets.'
Jo, mum of James and Daisy

'A step up from *Debenhams*, this café is a nice place to meet another parent, with baby, for a decent lunch on the riverside.'
Paige, mum of Miranda and Leo

Eating Out

Starbucks
Unit 3a North Street / Market Street
GU1 4LB
(01483) 504563
ukinfo@starbucks.com
www.starbucks.co.uk
[Alternative Starbucks venues – 195 High Street, GU1 3AW; 13-14 White Lion Walk, GU1 3DN; Burpham Sainsbury's, Clay Lane, GU4 7JU]

'Saturday mornings that include shopping in town have to be finished off with a coffee for Mummy and Daddy and a smoothie for William at *Starbucks*. We first went there when William was about four weeks old, and have been regular visitors to the (breastfeeding-friendly) upstairs sofas ever since. There can be a queue by late morning, but you can get cartons of smoothies, mini biscuits and chocolate shapes for little ones, and if you have a baby in tow, staff will happily provide hot water in large mugs for heating bottles.'
Claire, mum of William

Forum Restaurant
YMCA
Bridge Street
GU1 4SB
(01483) 532555 Ext. 510
catering@guildfordymca.org.uk
www.guildfordymca.org.uk

'The *YMCA* is very easy to access with a pram. The restaurant has views out over the river and you can either get a full hot meal or just a drink and a snack. I didn't see any high chairs but I suspect that they may well be available. There are pull-down changing facilities in the disabled toilet and breastfeeding was no problem. It is full of older people who like to coo at your baby!!'
Katy, mum of Edward

Pubs and Bars

The Black Swan
Old Lane
Ockham
KT11 1NG
(01932) 862364
blackswan@geronimo-inns.co.uk
www.geronimo-inns.co.uk/theblackswan

'We had a lovely meal here in pleasant surroundings with our baby asleep in her car seat. When we arrived the only seats available were in the bar, but the manager came over and offered us a table in the restaurant, as people hadn't turned up, and he thought we'd be more comfortable. There's a large outdoor eating area for warmer weather and we saw quite a few other mums with babies coming in just for coffee in the lounge area.'
Julie, mum of Ben and Katie

Brewers Fayre
The Parkway
Stoke Road
GU1 1UP
(01483) 450608
www.brewersfayre.co.uk

'We went on a weekday afternoon and were the only people in the place. They

are very child-friendly and promptly brought out a high chair and play pack with crayons. The children's menu would give Jamie Oliver heart failure, but our daughter was delighted with her rare treat of fish and chips. The food is exactly what you would expect, not fancy but cheap and hot. Sadly, *Brewers Fayre* has had to close all its outdoor play areas following unsupervised accidents at other branches.'
Jude, mum of Maia

Manor Inn Beefeater
Guildford Road
Godalming
GU7 3BX
(01483) 427134
www.beefeater.co.uk

'It has a good children's menu and the space inside is well structured. On warmer days, the children can play outside in the playground and if you wanted to burn up some calories after your meal it is possible to access the canal through the garden and go for a stroll along the river bank.'
Debra, mum of Ben and Eddie

The Mill at Elstead
Farnham Road
Elstead
GU8 6LE
(01252) 703333
http://www.function-rooms-uk.co.uk/cgi-bin/home.cgi

'Just prior to Christmas, we went for Sunday lunch to the restaurant with our then almost two-year-old, some friends and their toddler. There were lots of families and plenty of high chairs. Being a carvery, staff were happy for us to take our own bowls and cutlery for the children and the little ones ate from our plates. A baby with the family on the next table was doing this too – literally eating their roast and vegetables off the table and the staff didn't seem to mind the mess! The food was great and the desserts were lovely.

The location and grounds are very picturesque and there was a swan by the edge of the river as we were leaving that the kids were amused by. The staff were friendly and the toilets and changing facilities were good.'
Lisa, mum of Thomas

The Onslow Arms (l'auberge French restaurant)
The Street
West Clandon
GU4 7TE
(01483) 222447
onslowarms@massivepub.com
www.massivepub.com

'Although there are no baby-changing facilities, this is a very child-friendly pub. High chairs are available, and there's plenty of space on the floor in the ladies' to lay a changing mat out. When we asked for a children's portion of spaghetti without the meat sauce, the spaghetti was delightfully tossed in olive oil and herbs before having cheese sprinkled over it. It smelled divine. If you can't find something to tempt you on the pub menu, staff are happy to serve

food from the *L'auberge* restaurant menu in the pub dining areas.'
Fiona, mum of Thomas

The Parrot Inn
Forest Green
Dorking
RH5 5RZ
(01306) 621339

'The *Parrot Inn* is a country pub overlooking a large green, near Leith Hill. Oak beams and fireplaces give the place bags of atmosphere. There is a good range of beers and I have found the food and service consistently good over a number of visits. Lunch is served until 15.00 and it can get very busy so it's a good idea to book a table. The staff are friendly and there are changing facilities in the disabled toilet. The pub has ample parking, a beer garden, and its own farm shop selling a small range of produce.'
Louise, mum of James

The Percy Arms
75 Dorking Road
Chilworth
GU4 8NP
(01483) 561765
info.percy@tmp.uk.com
www.tailormadepub.co.uk/percy/default.php

'It is very family orientated and serves great food all week (although advance booking is recommended for weekends). My husband and I, with our son Jack, went there for Christmas lunch with our NCT friends. The staff were helpful and accommodating and were able to provide booster seats for all the babies. This pub/restaurant is great in the summer, too, with a large patio located to the rear.'
Becki, mum of Jack

'The *Percy Arms* is great for al fresco meals. There is a play area for kids, and decent, reasonable food. It is crammed on weekends, though.'
Paige, mum of Miranda and Leo

'This is a great pub for all sorts of occasions. Not only is the food great, but its beers have been awarded the Cask Marque. We first came across it on a sunny walk through the Surrey Hills, when we stopped in the large garden to quench our thirst and try the South African barbecued sausage. The tables are well spaced in the garden, so I've also found it easy to breastfeed discreetly. Inside there are several alcoves, large enough to fit a few babes in pushchairs to enjoy a long lunch after a walk over Blackheath. High chairs are available. There is a baby-changing table in the disabled toilet and a children's play area in the garden.'
Fiona, mum of Thomas

The Three Horseshoes
Dye House Rd
Thursley
Godalming
GU8 6QD
(01252) 703268

'We went here for our first meal out to celebrate my birthday nine days after

Thomas was born. We had a table at the edge of the patio, as I'd requested, so that I could breastfeed while facing away from other tables. The food is tasty, and real ale is available.

On other occasions we've enjoyed both after a pretty walk across Thursley Common. Weekend lunch-times are popular so I'd recommend booking. High chairs are available. There is a baby-changing table in the disabled toilet.'
Fiona, mum of Thomas

The Weyside
Millbrook
GU1 3XJ
(01483) 568024
weyside@pubexplorer.com
http://pub-explorer.com/surrey/pub/weysideguildford.htm

'This is always a nice place to go when it's sunny. You can incorporate a walk by the river before or after lunch. Two high chairs available, but no changing facilities.'
Leena, mum of Ella

The White Hart
The Green
Pirbright
GU24 0LP
(01483) 799715

'*The White Hart* is a great place to take babies/toddlers. Staff are really helpful and the food is fantastic. There is a lovely garden and it is very welcoming and peaceful. A must for Sunday lunch!'
Avril, mum of Scarlett

'This is a 17th century tavern offering excellent food and drink in comfortable surroundings. The menu is mostly modern English and is well presented and tasty. The venue is cosy and inviting; all staff are polite and friendly. Little extra touches such as pistachio nuts brought to your table make the experience pleasurable.

It has a large beer garden with a patio area, which is great for families with older children. Families with babies/toddlers may struggle if their child is not keen to sit on laps or in a pushchair as there is only one high chair available. If possible, go after the Sunday lunch rush. It is a great place to sit outdoors enjoying the sunshine with family/friends or be cosy inside with the fire.'
Anna, mum of Logan

The White Horse
Middle Street
Shere
GU5 9HS
(01483) 202518
whitehorse.shere@pubexplorer.com
www.pub-explorer.com/surrey/pub/whitehorseshere.htm

'*The White Horse* is our favourite pub for a family Sunday lunch. Shere itself is incredibly pretty so we always combine our lunch with a walk. The pub opens at noon, and as long as we arrive promptly we've never had a problem finding a space. We usually go to the little room up the step towards the back of the pub. You can usually squeeze two families around the big table at one end. The menu is

good, prices are reasonable and we've always had excellent service.'
Jo, mum of Thomas, George and Rebecca

The Seahorse
52-54 The Street
Shalford
GU4 8BU
(01483) 514351

'Occasionally we park at The Seahorse, grab lunch, and walk along the tow path up to the toy shops in Shalford and back again. It is a great way to spend lunchtime. Although there are no high chairs, when it's quiet you can spread out and take in mobile high chairs.

We usually meet up with five mums and babies and the staff are quick and helpful and the food is great!'
Avril, mum of Scarlett

The Stoke Pub & Pizzeria
103 Stoke Road
GU1 4JN
(01483) 504296

'We love it here. The pizzas are freshly made and delicious. You can order six-inch pizzas for under £3.00, ideal for little ones. Although there is no children's area as such, there is comfortable seating. It is near Stoke Park and there are picnic benches outside for summer days.'
Thora, mum of Freyja

'Highly recommended. You can watch the pizzas being freshly made, and the dough balls are the best! The pizzas have interesting toppings, such as Peking Duck, and are good value for money. There is generally a good atmosphere in here. You tend to see lots of families early evening, you can sit outside with your children, although there is no garden *per se*.'
Richard, dad of Roald and Seth

Worplesdon Place Country Pub and Dining
Perry Hill
Worplesdon
GU3 3RY
(01483) 232407
www.worplesdonplacepub.co.uk

'Since being refurbished at the end of 2006, it has really improved. The food is 100% better and the staff are really helpful and quick. Children are always welcomed. There are high chairs and child portions of most main course meals. We have been there a few times recently with friends and a few children and have been very impressed!'
Avril, mum of Scarlett

'This rather grand looking pub/restaurant is actually a very child-friendly place to eat. There is an extensive beer garden with a duck pond (fish and duck food can be purchased!) and plenty of space to run about.

The staff are friendly and helpful with children and provide high chairs and a limited but home-cooked children's menu. The food is delicious and it is great to be able to eat in such nice surroundings for the same price as our favourite town

centre pizzeria! There is a baby-changing table in the disabled toilet.'
Heather, mum of Tom

Takeaways

Bamboo Garden (Chinese)
13 Guildford Park Road
GU2 7NA
(01483) 560361
Open: Tues – Thurs 5.00 – 11.30 pm;
Fri – Sat 5.00 pm – 12.00 am;
Sun 6.00 – 11.00 pm. No credit cards.

'Located opposite the back entrance to Guildford train station, the *Bamboo Garden* is the ideal commuter takeaway! When baby ensured that cooking an evening meal was impossible, I'd call my husband on the train and ask him to pick up supper on his way home! Lots of choice at reasonable prices, including omelette and chips for something simple.'
Julie, mum of Ben and Katie

Bombay Spice Restaurant (Indian)
17 Park Street
GU1 4XB
(01483) 454272
(01483) 454568
Open daily: 12.00 – 3.00 pm;
6.00 – 11.30 pm

'A nice Indian restaurant to eat in, if you ever get a night off without the kids, but it also does great takeaways. We always phone ahead with our order and it's usually ready for collection within half an hour. Menu contains all the usual range of Indian dishes, so even if you don't have a menu to hand, you can order your favourite and the staff are pretty sure to be able to cook it for you. Word of warning – don't park in the office car park off The Mount, behind the restaurant. It warns that they clamp and we found out that they mean it – even at night!'
Julie, mum of Ben and Katie

Chopsticks (Chinese)
4 Stoughton Road
Bellfields
GU1 1LL
(01483) 538789
Open daily: 12.00 – 2.00 pm; 4.30 – 10.00 pm

'This is a fantastic Cantonese take away, whose staff now know us by name!! Home delivery is available for an additional £1.00, and the service is swift. Strongly recommended.'
Heather, mum of Jessica

Fish and Chips
83 Stoke Road
GU1 4HT
(01483) 561671
Open daily: 11.30 am – 2.00 pm;
5.00 – 11.00 pm

'This fish and chip shop is tiny, but does some of the best fish and chips and pies I have tasted, and at lower prices than other places. Parking is a bit of a pain though, unless you can park in the pub car park next door.'
Maggie, mum of Alice and Katy

'We use this fish bar a lot. It's very good value for money, and you get fast service. The portion sizes aren't bad and the food is very well cooked.'
Richard, dad of Roald and Seth

Guildford Kebab House (Turkish)
11 Epsom Road
GU1 3JT
(01483) 534780
Open: Sun, Tues, Wed 12.00 pm – 1.00 am;
Mon, Thurs, Fri, Sat 12.00 pm – 3.00 am

'The Turkish kebabs are tasty and huge, although you do have to wait as they are cooked to order.'
Maggie, mum of Alice and Katy

Ho Ho Chinese takeaway
38 Barrack Rd
Stoughton
GU2 9RU
(01483) 566405
Open: Tues – Sat 12.00 – 2.00 pm; 5.00 – 11.00 pm; Sun 6.00 – 11.00 pm.

'*HoHo* is one of the best Chinese takeaways we've ever found, everything on the menu is great (and we've tasted most of it!!). I've even eaten from there while pregnant and it was the first thing we had after having coming home from the hospital too! It's best to call in your order as it will only ever take '10 minutes', which is just long enough to finish a glass of wine. Then you can go and collect, and the prawn crackers are still warm when we get home. Enjoy.'
Jenny, mum of Imogen and Harrison

India
86 Haydon Place
GU1 4LR
(01483) 459331
Open daily: 12.00 – 2.00 pm and 5.30 – 11.30 pm

'When we first moved to Guildford we tried out several Indian takeaways and this was far and away my favourite. The dishes contain real meat and vegetables with tasty sauces and spices (as opposed to insipid squares of unidentifiable material floating in a sea of indifferent sauce).'
Tessa, mum of Daisy, Zach and Jake

Kohinoor Tandoori Restaurant
24 Woodbridge Road
GU1 1DY
(01483) 306051
info@kohinoorguildford.com
www.kohinoorguildford.com
Open daily: 12.00 – 2.30 pm and 6.00 – 11.30 pm

'This is our favourite takeaway – the Balti dishes are fantastic. We ate here quite often when I was pregnant and lived in the flats across the street (unfortunately the hot curries failed to bring on labour!) and started getting takeaways after we had Audrey. The staff are very friendly; my husband enjoys letting them fuss over him while he waits for them to prepare our order – always fast, hot and delicious!'
Kelley, mum of Audrey

'If we want an Indian takeaway, this is the one we use. The food is tasty and

Eating Out

plentiful. The preparation time is usually about 20 minutes, which I think is fairly standard for Indian takeaways.

It is also a restaurant with an 'eat as much as you like' buffet on Sundays, but we have not yet tried this.'
Kay, mum of Alex, Brian and Theo

Miah's Takeaway (Indian)
139 Worplesdon Road
GU2 9XA
(01483) 454540 / 454560
info@miahtakeaway.co.uk
www.miahtakeaway.co.uk
Open daily 5.30 – 11.00 pm

'The takeaway offers a good selection of very tasty dishes from the Indian and Bangladeshi cuisine. The staff are very friendly and are prepared to take orders for meals that are not included on the menu.

For orders over £12.00 the takeaway offers free delivery within five miles, or a 10% discount if collected.'
Dimitra, mum of Electra

Oriental Express (Chinese)
11-13 Madrid Road,
GU2 7NU
(01483) 453838
Open daily: Mon – Sat 12.00 – 2.00 pm; 5.00 – 11.00 pm; Sun 5.00 – 10.00 pm

'This Chinese takeaway does substantial tasty dishes. The service has always been quick and friendly. We used to live close enough that you could pick up a takeaway on the walk home. Now we have moved to the other side of town, but we still drive across to use this one.'
Kay, mum of Alex, Brian and Theo

'We really like this Chinese. There is a good selection of food, which is really nicely cooked and still hot when we get it home, the service is prompt, efficient and friendly, and the prices reasonable. What more could you ask for? Oh, of course, the delicious complementary prawn crackers that arrive with every order.'
Emma, mum of Charlotte and Louis

Purbani (Indian)
98 Stoke Road
GU1 4JN
(01483) 579292
Open daily: 5.30 – 11.30 pm

'This Indian takeaway does some excellent lamb and veggie dishes. The service is friendly and you are in and out within 20 minutes. Good value for money.'
Richard, dad of Roald and Seth

Red Rose (Indian)
2 Bellfields Road
GU1 1QG
(01483) 455655 / 455773
www.redroseguildford.com
Open daily: 6.00 – 11.30 pm
Free home delivery within four miles.

'One of the best curry houses in Surrey. Gorgeous fresh authentic food. Great fish and vegetarian options. You can even ask the chef to make each dish hotter or

Eating Out

milder as your taste buds desire. The service is brilliant whether you eat in the restaurant, collect your takeaway or have it delivered.'
Bally, mum of Jasmine and Saffron

Ripley Curry Garden Indian Cuisine
High Street
Ripley
GU23 6AY
(01483) 224153
Open daily: 12.00 – 2.00 pm;
5.30 – 11.30 pm

'Ripley *Curry Garden* does excellent takeaways, and we travel here rather than to our more local Indian takeaway/restaurant.'
Maggie, mum of Alice and Katy

Seafare (Fish and Chips)
206 London Road   147 Worplesdon Road
Burpham   Stoughton
GU4 7JS   GU2 9XA
(01483) 534253   (01483) 562547
Open: Mon – Sat 11.30 am – 2.00 pm; 5.00 – 11.00 pm; Sun: Burpham closed; Stoughton 5.00 – 11.00 pm

'Winner of various regional best fish and chips restaurants over the years. As a Northerner and therefore an expert on 'chippies', I would definitely recommend them. Big portions too. Could only be improved by the addition of gravy to the menu. They do kids meal deals that include a toy and drink.'
Helen, mum of Dominic and Laura

Shangri-La (Oriental)
7 Kingpost Parade
London Road
Burpham
GU1 1YP
(01483) 502778 / (07816) 047258
Open: Tues – Thurs 5.00 – 10.30 pm; Fri – Sat 5.00 – 11.00 pm; Sun 5.00 – 10.30 pm. Collection only. No credit cards.

'Good selection of quickly prepared Peking, Szechuan, Thai and Chinese food, and even Japanese noodles. There is an open kitchen so you can see your order being cooked. We have enjoyed everything we have ordered from there. Our favourites include Shredded Beef, Duck, Chop Suey, and Special Fried Rice. There is also a handy cashpoint and an off-licence in the same parade of shops.'
Helen, mum of Dominic and Laura

'A varied menu of Chinese and Thai food, so good that everyone can find something. The noodle selection is fantastic. You have to collect but service is really quick and the food still piping hot at home.'
Bally, mum of Jasmine and Saffron

Thai Takeaway at the Ship Inn
Worplesdon Road
Pitch Place
GU3 3LB
(01483) 237311
Open: Tues – Sat 12.00 – 3.00 pm; 6.00 – 10.00 pm; Sun 12.00 – 8.00pm

'We love the Thai food at the *Ship Inn*. The set meal for two is great value, and

we always have spring rolls left over for packed lunches the next day. I particularly love the sweet and sour fish, and chicken phad Thai, and although you have to collect, my husband says that is fine as he gets to eat the complimentary prawn crackers on the way home while I'm putting William to bed (and yes they do know us by name – shame on my home cooking skills!) Great for any days you get home from work and childcare runs, and discover there is nothing in the fridge.'
Claire, mum of William

Tong Tong (Chinese)
28 Woodbridge Road
GU1 1ED
(01483) 562205
Open: Sun, Mon, Wed, Thurs 5.00 – 11.00pm; Fri, Sat 12.00 – 2.00 pm; 5.00 – 11.30 pm. No credit cards.

'The service here is generally quick and friendly. It has a fairly reasonable selection of food, which is not bad at all.'
Richard, dad of Roald and Seth

Wagamama (Oriental)
25-29 High Street
GU1 3DY
(01483) 457779
www.wagamama.com
[Note: there is a fun kids' 'Noodle-Doodlers' page on the website]
Open daily: Mon – Fri 12.00 – 11.00 pm; Sat 11.30 am – 11.00 pm; Sun 12.00 – 10.00 pm

'If you're prepared to go and pick it up, a takeaway from *Wagamama* makes a nice change and is a bit of a cut above standard takeaway food. It does hot Japanese dishes, mainly noodles in soup or sauce or cooked on a griddle, and there are also some rice dishes and a couple of salads, plus starters. It also does some interesting fresh fruit juices.'
Tessa, mum of Daisy, Zach and Jake

'Unusually, *Wagamama* has a children's menu that is also available for takeaway! Nice for something a bit different.'
Emma, mum of Charlotte and Louis

7
Services

Victoria Jackson

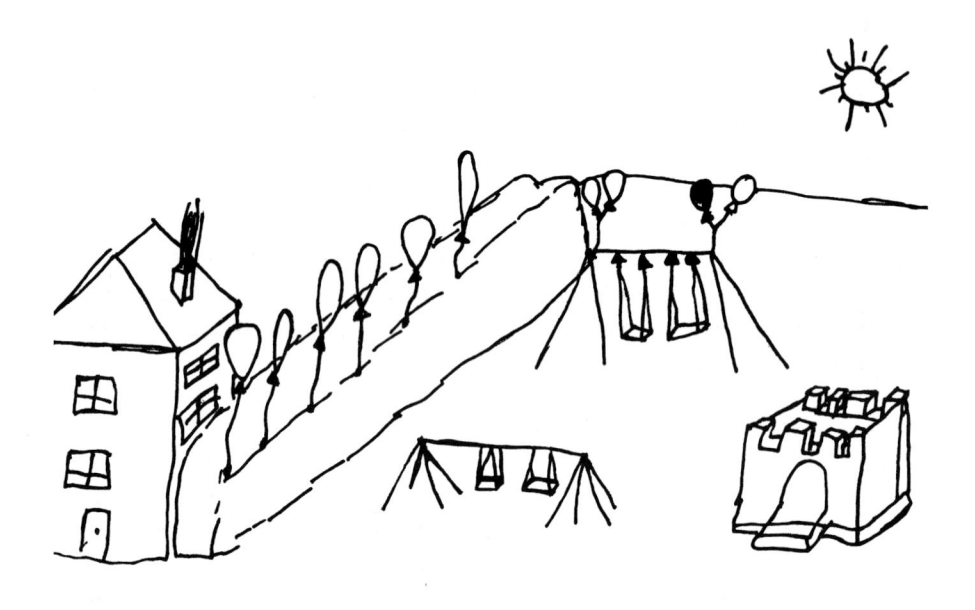

With the arrival of children you suddenly enter a new world of things you didn't know you needed. No sooner have you learned to fold your pushchair than you're on to the wonderful world of children's parties. Whether you do it yourself at home or take over a venue, Guildford offers plenty of specialist shops, businesses and venues to help. Where can you get your children's hair cut? Do you want it to be a quick 'in-and-out' before they get bored, or an exciting event with distractions and a souvenir lock of hair for the album? And thinking of albums, how do you find a photographer who's good with children?

If you're feeling green, washable nappies are another mystery until you look into the possibilities. *Guildford Borough Council* is increasingly supporting the idea, and below are recommendations from enthusiastic mothers who have each found a brand, a supplier or a compromise that suits both them and their babies.

Don't forget *Guildford Library*, an invaluable asset right in the middle of the town, above all for books but also for information and events (see *'Things to do'* for the very popular 'Baby Bounce and Rhyme' sessions (p46) and 'Guildford Library Storytime' (p59). The *Tourist Office* is bulging with information both local and further afield. Details of these and other sources of information are listed below.

Parties

If you can't face holding a birthday party at home, can't fit in all your children's friends or want a different kind of party adventure for your child, there are plenty of alternatives. Church halls are a well-tried option and you can do your own catering, while a soft play venue gives you a ready-made activity and can provide food.

The venues in the selection below have been recommended specifically as being good for party venues, but it's worth looking also at the *Things to do* and *Places to visit* chapters for other possibilities. We've also included a selection of party suppliers that are useful whether you're at home or somewhere more exotic, providing everything from birthday cake candles to bouncy castles.

Venues

All Saints Church Hall
Vicarage Gate
Onslow Village
GU2 7QJ
(01483) 565306 (Mr and Mrs Reed)
www.allsaintschurchgfd.org.uk

'Good-sized hall, can enquire about hiring or using the playgroup's toys. Book well ahead, affordable prices for hall hire.'
Helen, mum of Dominic and Laura

'A great party venue, especially in the summer when you can also make use of the field behind the hall. The kitchen and loos have recently been refurbished, which is good but means the price has gone up too – it's now £40 per session. It is a reasonably sized, clean hall, with children's tables and chairs, a well-stocked kitchen and parking for several cars. Book well in advance because it is a popular venue!'
Jo, mum of Thomas, George and Rebecca

Farncombe Fun Zone
(formerly the **Cool Club**)
The Warehouse
Owen Road
Godalming
GU7 3AY
(01483) 861666
[See main entry on p39 '*Things to do*'.]

'Freyja had her second birthday party here and we have been to many there since. Definitely worth it for those looking to 'outsource' their child's birthday party. Prices are reasonable.'
Thora, mum of Freyja

Services

Guildford Methodist Church Hall
Woodbridge Road (entrance side door on Wharf Road)
GU1 4RG
(01483) 564300
www.guildfordmethodist.org

'There is a spacious upstairs hall with a kitchen which is a great space for parties. There is a toddler group which meets there on Tuesdays, the *Getaway Club* (p14). Great toys are stored off this room. If you get prior permission you may be able to hire the toys for the party.'
Helen, mum of Dominic and Laura

Gym Jams
Normandy Village Hall
Manor Fruit Farm
Glaziers Lane
Normandy
GU3 2DE
(01932) 340379 (Barry or Millie)
info@gym-jams.co.uk
www.gym-jams.co.uk
[See main entry on p40 'Things to do'.]

'*Gym Jams* is available for hire for private parties on either a Wednesday afternoon (approx £75.00) or the weekend (approx £125) and is fabulous for one to three-year-olds. We had twenty-five toddlers bouncing and running around for an hour and a half. All the soft play equipment, ball pit and bouncy castle are set up for you; tea/coffee-making facilities are available within the hire prices, and you can bring party food and cakes and decorations. We also hired a face-painter who was fabulous at keeping the kids occupied, and the slightly older toddlers loved showing off their faces to everyone.'
Jenny, mum of Imogen and Harrison

'We had a party for four-year-olds and they all had a fantastic time. The large hall was filled with soft play equipment ranging from a ball pool, see-saw, huge building blocks, slide and a bouncy castle. Although much of the equipment was probably more ideally suited to crawlers and toddlers (e.g. soft toys on play mats enclosed by a soft low novelty wall), this didn't stop the older children from thoroughly enjoying themselves – they threw all the balls out of the pool and flung them round the room, filled the pool with soft building blocks, charged round the hall with the hoop-la and used up their last scraps of energy on the bouncy castle. They then sat down to eat for a well-earned rest at a long party table. Chairs and covered tables were provided and we brought along all the other tableware, food, party bags, balloons etc., and we had full use of the very well-equipped kitchen (which includes a huge fridge, an urn for

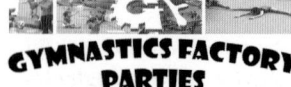

GYMNASTICS FACTORY PARTIES
Action packed parties for all!
Preschool parties (2-4yrs)
with parent
Gym'll Fix It Parties (5-10yrs)
up to 18 children
Full Monty Parties (5-10yrs)
up to 24 children - every aspect catered for!
FOR DETAILS CALL
01483 455 060
OR CHECK OUT
www.gymnasticsfactory.co.uk

teas/coffees and a dishwasher). Although the hall is only a few years old, there are sadly no baby-changing facilities in the toilets. However, *Gym Jams* can provide changing mats for use in the hall. The parties are limited to 25 children under the age of five and last for two hours plus a little setting up and dismantling time. They cost around £120.00 and get booked up months in advance as the hall is used for lots of different activities. There is ample parking.'
Miranda, mum of Kieron and Anthony

Gymnastics Factory
Pew Corner
Old Portsmouth Road
GU3 1LP
(01483) 459703
info@gymnasticsfactory.co.uk
www.gymnasticsfactory.co.uk
[See also p23 and p65 'Things to do'.]

'My five-year-old daughter and eight-year-old son had an excellent joint party at the *Gymnastics Factory*. The experienced, energetic and fun-loving coaches kept 24 children entertained with games, races and a circuit of the amazing gym facilities, including the trampoline, trapeze, foam pit, bars, beam and vaults. This was followed by party food and drinks that were included in the party price. The only thing we had to do was bring a cake and party bags. All the children had a fantastic time and talked about the party for days afterwards. We've already booked another party for next year!'
Jo, mum of Cerys and Thomas

The Herons Swimming and Fitness Centre
Kings Road
Haslemere
GU27 2QT
(01428) 658484
enquiries@theheronsswimandfitnesscentre.co.uk
www.dcleisurecentres.co.uk
[See main entry on p34 'Things to do'.]

'We tried the bouncy castle and soft play party (food provided) – a big success.'
Nicki, mum of George and Olivia

Lord Pirbright's Hall
Pirbright Green
Guildford Road
Pirbright
GU24 0JT
(01483) 476432 (hire)
www.parish-council.com/Pirbright

'A nice hall with a separate kitchen and eating area, and a playground next to it.'
Tessa, mum of Daisy, Zach and Jake

Merrow Methodist Church Hall
Bushy Hill Drive
Merrow
GU4 7XR
(01483) 537655 (church)

'Lots of space and separate areas for play and party tables. Very reasonable hire rates. Book well in advance. Leave message if you get answerphone. Has its own car park at the back.'
Helen, mum of Dominic and Laura

Services

Onslow Village Hall
Wilderness Road
Onslow Village
GU2 7QR
(07771) 546009 (Angela Joule)

'Since I took over bookings in March 2007, we have seen an increase in the number of children's bookings. Everybody has been very pleased, and all comments favourable. The hall, which is a good size, costs £12.00 per hour, and includes a well-equipped kitchen and its own car park. You can negotiate use of small tables and chairs with the playgroup.'
Angela Joule, hall bookings coordinator

Rainbow Tots
Knaphill Scout Hall
Waterers Rise
Knaphill
GU21 2HU
(07803) 600720 (Angela Sanderson)
(07885) 702414 (Hazel)
info@rainbowtots.com
www.rainbowtots.com
[See main review on p41 'Things to do'.]

'I recently held my daughter's third birthday party here. Fantastic – it was so easy! The venue was perfect, offering facilities for both birthday guests and their younger siblings. The food was super (fresh and healthy) and much enjoyed. Tea-time was the only quiet time that we had! I would recommend *Rainbow Tots* to anyone looking for a stress-free fun party for their toddlers. We will be back!'
Holly, mum of Freya

St Catherine's Village Hall
Chestnut Avenue
GU2 4DW
(01483) 568001 (Mrs A Bailey)

'The hall provided an excellent venue for my daughter's fourth birthday, with plenty of space for games, running around and for parents who stayed to watch. Tables and chairs for small children were available and could be set up in a separate room situated between the main hall and the kitchen. Facilities in the kitchen were reasonable but it would be worth checking that what you need is supplied. Take your own tea towels, baking trays etc. Toilets were fine and plenty of parking. Morning and afternoon sessions cost £20.00.'
Gillie, mum of Lily and Marcus

---

mucky pups
where kids have messy fun and we clean up !!!

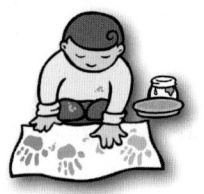

Contact Kim or Charli for details of classes in your area

07852 606142

www.mucky-pups.com
we are a member of the Preschool Learning Alliance

Services

St Mark's Church Hall (Wyke)
Guildford Road
Normandy
GU3 2DA
(01483) 235923 (Ted Valler)
www.stmarkswyke.co.uk

'This hall is only a few years old and is a nice venue for a party, with space for a bouncy castle, running around and a party table. Little tables and chairs are available for use at parties. There is also a well-equipped kitchen with a serving hatch into the hall, plus toilets (including a nappy-changing table) and plenty of parking. Booking details and prices are on the notice-board outside; a whole afternoon costs from around £40.00.'
Miranda, mum of Kieron and Anthony

St Pius' Church Hall
Laustan Close (off Horseshoe Lane East)
Merrow
GU1 2TS
(01483) 572605

'Reasonable rates, with good kitchen facilities and large well-lit hall.'
Sonya, mum of Eleanor and Charles

West Horsley Village Hall
The Street
West Horsley
KT24 6DD
(01483) 285454 (Mrs B Sansom)
www.westhorsley.info

'Two rooms for hire: both have kitchen facilities and toilets, reasonable rates – approx £7.00 per hour for the smaller of the two, the Cedar room. The larger room has a stage. Adjacent to newly refurbished West Horsley playground.'
Vicki, mum of George and Finlay

YMCA Midwey House
Wharf Road
GU1 4RP
(01483) 565969

'A nice venue for children's or grown-ups' parties. Has well-appointed kitchen with lots of cups, plates, cutlery, etc. (just remember to wash up afterwards). An entrance room can be used to set up tables for kids' food and separate modern hall for the party activities. Lots of folding tables and chairs there to use. Hire available for the day or half-day at competitive rates. So long as there is no other function booked that day (check just before your event) there is no pressure to arrive or get out by a certain time so you can get ready and clear up in your own time. Make sure it is clear on the invitation that it is Wharf Road YMCA and not the town centre YMCA.'
Helen, mum of Dominic and Laura

Party Equipment Hire

Boing Bouncy Castles
(08456) 445569
www.boingcastles.com

'We hired an octopus bouncy castle for Dominic's third birthday. It was October and after an hour of happy bouncing the

heavens opened and it poured down. We had ordered one with a roof just in case, which did allow another fifteen minutes of bouncing in the rain before it started to get a bit water-logged! The staff were very helpful and friendly; they came over early to set up in our garden and let us keep the castle till 6.00 pm. They have a very wide range of castles and other bouncy things for hire.'
Helen, mum of Dominic and Laura

'We ordered the *'Dinoslide'* for Charlotte's third birthday, mostly because it was in her favourite pink and purple colours. It was wonderful; we had a garden full of very young children bouncing and sliding for two hours – a very easy way to host a party. Even though we got to keep it for the whole day, Charlotte and Louis weren't bored by the time the party guests arrived, and in fact, were sad to see it leave when it was finally removed at 6.00 pm.'
Emma, mum of Charlotte and Louis

Farncombe Fun Zone
(formerly the **Cool Club**)
The Warehouse
Owen Road
Godalming
GU7 3AY
(01483) 861666
[Ssee also p39 *'Things to do'* and p167 'Party venues']

'The *Fun Zone* has recently started to hire out a range of bouncy castles. Worth checking out.'
Helen, mum of Dominic and Laura

Godalming Toy Library
Broadwater Park Community Centre
Summers Road
Godalming
GU7 3BH
01483 424307 (Kirsten)
www.surreycc.gov.uk
Open every Tuesday (including holidays)
2.00 – 4.00 pm
[See main review under 'Information Centres' below p188]

'Can hire toys for two weeks at reasonable prices. Why not hire them for parties? A wide range of toys available, including large outdoor toys.'
Helen, mum of Dominic and Laura

Party Accessories

Apache Tears
19 White Lion Walk
GU1 3DN
(01483) 457874
info@apachetears.co.uk
www.apachetears.co.uk

'For an unusual party bag that won't get tossed aside immediately, try *Apache*

Godalming Toy Library

Open all year round. Every Tuesday from 2:00-3:30pm
Broadwater Park Community Centre, Summers Lane, Farncombe
(next to the Leisure Centre)
Contact Kirsten 07887963606 for further information

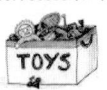

Fantastic selection of large and small toys to rent out. Children can play in our spacious hall or in the garden in good weather. Free parking! Parents, grandparents and carers of pre-school children welcome. Membership £8 a year.

Tears. Along with crystals, chimes, prints of unicorns in starlight and other 'new age' paraphernalia, there is a selection of small, polished, semi-precious stones of various colours, all about the size of a pound coin.

For my daughter's party guests, I put four different stones into a pretty organza drawstring pouch (also available at *Apache Tears*). They were like jewels wrapped up in silk, and the girls treasured them. Even better – each bag and stones only cost about £2.00! Beats the same old plastic tat by a mile!'

Kris, mum of Olivia and Victoria

Party Pieces
Childs Court Farm
Ashampstead Common
Reading
RG8 7BR
(01635) 201844
sales@partypieces.co.uk
www.partypieces.co.uk

'This mail-order company for 'children's parties by post' has everything for themed parties from pirates and princesses, to *Disney* and *CBeebies* characters – there's a huge selection. You can order all tableware, loads of party game ideas, party bag gifts, etc.

I think one of the best products are the party trays; these come in many different fun designs and incorporate box, scoop (for food), napkin, cup/straw – just pile up each with party food and drink and you are done!'

Helen, mum of Dominic and Laura

Partyland
17 Princes Mead Shopping Centre
Farnborough
GU14 6YB
(01252) 370100

'*Partyland* has a fantastic range of party accessories, well worth the trip to Farnborough, great value prices. It is also next door to *Asda*, where you can buy the party food.

Just around the corner from *Wizzy World* [see main entry under '*Things to do*' p44]; I leave the kids here with hubby while I shop!'

Helen, mum of Dominic and Laura

Special Occasions
Fairlands Post Office
57 Fairlands Avenue
GU3 3NB
(01483) 236200

'*Special Occasions* is a hidden gem. You can get everything for your party including invitations, cards, decorations, banners and party bags. Helium balloons can be pre-ordered to pick up on the day or day before. There is a great range of pocket-money-priced party bag fillers. There are novelty cake tins for hire, cake decorations, boards and boxes.

We love the 'Dominic' and 'Laura' cake candles, each letter is a candle, and good value as we reuse them each birthday! There is also a wide variety of adults' and children's fancy dress, face paints, wigs and so forth.'

Helen, mum of Dominic and Laura

Services

Entertainers

Smartie Artie
(01582) 600529; (0870) 3500529
enquiries@smartieartie.co.uk
www.smartieartie.com

'We had *Smartie Artie* number 11' for Dominic's fourth birthday. He was hilarious, and kept over 20 four-year-olds enthralled for two hours; he was also an expert in crowd control, just what was needed.

For the first hour *Smartie Artie* does a funny magic show, then he helps give out the food at the birthday tea. The second hour consists of party games, including pass the parcel, musical bumps, etc. He provides the prizes. All you have to do is the food and party bags. Let somebody else take the strain of entertaining the little darlings.

Dominic's sides were aching from laughing so much by the end; he had also been made to feel like a very special party boy.'
Helen, mum of Dominic and Laura

Tumble Tots
(01483) 420741
www.tumbletots.com
[See main entry on p25 '*Things to do*'.]

'Party entertainment is provided for two hours for up to twenty-five children. For the first hour children take turns over a supervised obstacle course. After a refuel break for tea, there are party games, including a parachute. This party will really tire the children out. My two kids had a great time. Great party music on throughout. The facilitators are friendly, very experienced, keep everybody in order, and great fun. All kids love them.'
Helen, mum of Dominic and Laura

Catering Equipment Hire

Alexander Taylor Cakes
20 Woodbridge Road
GU1 1DY
(01483) 566661
info@alexandertaylorcakes.co.uk
www.alexandertaylorcakes.co.uk

'As well as making cakes for any occasion, this shop is a treasure-trove of accessories for decorating and making cakes. It also hires out cake tins of many shapes and designs such as numbers, super-heroes, and so forth.'
Helen, mum of Dominic and Laura

The Farmhouse Kitchen
Crown Court
High Street
Godalming
GU7 1DY
(01483) 860424

'I love this little shop; it's 'gadget heaven' and there is nothing you can't find for your kitchen in here. Regarding kids' parties you can hire novelty cake tins, and there is an array of accessories for decorating your own cakes – you can make them as easy or difficult as you like!'
Emma, mum of Charlotte and Louis

Hairdressers

You may be skilled or brave enough to cut your children's hair for a while, but if they rebel at the pudding-basin, here is a selection of kindly hairdressers to make the experience painless and even fun.

D's Hair Salon
Wilderness Road
Onslow Village
GU2 7QR
(01483) 573588

'Cheapest quality kids' haircuts in the area. Rebecca is very friendly and there are books and a special chair for kids to sit in. However, no pushchairs allowed in as the place is small, so not great if you also have a baby with you.'
Paige, mum of Miranda and Leo

Haircontacts
22 Woodbridge Road
GU1 1DY
(01483) 532861
www.haircontacts.co.uk

'I have had my hair cut here with baby on lap/in pram/in arms of spare member of staff. Also take son to barber's at the back (no appointment, wait your turn), and daughter to ladies' section for her first haircut (lock of hair provided in an envelope for memento). Best thing is the playroom, like a den, with great collection of *Lego*, crayons, cuddly toys, etc.'
Helen, mum of Dominic and Laura

Jack's of London
165 High Street
GU1 3AJ
(01483) 531406
guildford@jacksoflondon.co.uk
www.jacksoflondon.co.uk

'The first couple of times I took William to the hairdressers, it was a bit of a disaster, until I found *Jack's* – this is a barber's in the high street, which has televisions showing sport and offers drinks to the adults, plus has lollipops to bribe toddlers to be good while their hair is being cut.

William has now been three times, and is excellent at sitting still while the friendly assistants get on with his short back and sides while Mummy and Daddy have a coffee. Only faults are that they are so quick, I haven't finished a cup of coffee yet! Cuts are cheaper in the week for little ones than at the weekend.'
Claire, mum of William

Martin G
traditional barber
22 Woodbridge Road, Guildford Surrey, GU1 1DY
www.haircontacts.co.uk
(01483) 532 282
opening hours
monday   closed
tuesday   08.30 – 17.30
wednesday   08.30 – 17.30
thursday   08.30 – 19.00
friday   08.30 – 19.00
saturday   08.30 – 16.00
appointments not necessary

Services

Kerry's Hair Design
2 Kingfisher Court
Kingfisher Drive
Merrow Park
GU4 7EW
(01483) 536780

'The staff are great with children and we've always come out with a good hair cut.'
Sally, mum of James

Niki's Hairdressers
81 Stoke Road
GU1 4HT
(01483) 440444
Special rates for under-10s on Wednesday and Thursday – girls £13.50; boys £10.00

'No chairs shaped like aeroplanes or certificates for first haircuts here, just a small, friendly hairdresser who will give your little one a good haircut.'
Louise, mum of James

Spikes and Curls
61a Downing Street
Farnham
GU9 7PN
(01252) 711121
info@spikesandcurls.com
www.spikesandcurls.com

'We just love going to *Spikes and Curls*. When my son needed his first haircut, I had trouble finding a hairdresser that cuts hair for very small children until I came across *Spikes and Curls*. Noah was strapped into a toy car and was playing while he had his hair cut. We were even given a certificate including a lock of hair and a photo.

When the little ones are very scared they can sit on mum's lap and the hairdressers tend to offer raisins as a distraction. There are plenty of toys there and my son cries when he has to leave. For the older children there are also distractions around – each seat is fitted with a TV showing children's DVDs.'
Nadine, mum of Noah and Luca

'*Spikes and Curls* is a dedicated children's hairdresser, specifically designed for children; it provides little chairs, TV screens playing *CBeebies*, *Shrek*, etc. to occupy your little one during his/her haircut, a waiting area with toys and a little table and chairs, and an offer of raisins or a lollipop when it is all over.

I was delighted to find *Spikes and Curls* because my son was eighteen months old and my hairdressing skills were no longer capable of keeping his hair under control. I remember on his first visit he was more than happy to sit in the specially adapted old-fashioned fire-engine ringing the bell during his haircut.

The staff are used to children that move all the time and he wasn't expected to keep still; the final result was a very nice professional cut. We have continued to go every couple of months and watched the most challenging tots have their hair cut from those that scream, to those that want to sit on mum's knee and all end up with lovely haircuts.'
Irene, mum of Joe

Haircontacts

22, Woodbridge Road, Guildford, Surrey, GU1 1DY
www.haircontacts.co.uk
(01483) 532 861

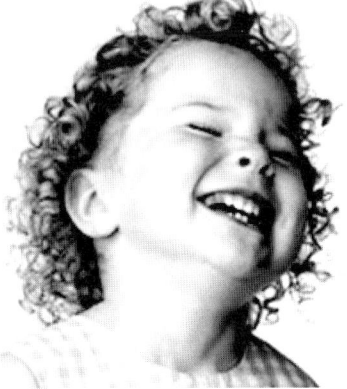

opening hours

Monday	closed
Tuesday	08:30 – 17:30
Wednesday	08:30 – 17:30
Thursday	08:30 – 19:00
Friday	08:30 – 19:00
Saturday	08:30 – 16:30

Our aim at Haircontacts is to provide all our customers, both adult & child a high quality service in a fun and friendly environment.

We have a children's play room filled with toys and activities that your little ones can play with while you relax and enjoy the comfort of our professional stylists.

Late night opening hours are designed so visits can be made to suit parents' hectic lifestyles.

With our children's play room and a safe and friendly environment children and adults will love to come. Every child goes away with a lollypop and a smile.

Appointments are recommended

Services

Trotters
Unit 6 White Lion Walk
GU1 3DN
01483 454 668
enquiry@trotters.co.uk
www.trotters.co.uk

'In addition to selling clothes, shoes, toys etc. for children, *Trotters* specialises in children's hairdressing with a large aquarium to keep children entranced while they sit.'
Emma, mum of Charlotte and Louis

Photographers

You'll have hundreds of snaps of your children but sometimes nothing beats a professional shot, whether an individual child or a memento of the whole family, a studio portrait or a more 'candid' picture of your child at play.

Castle Studios
40-42 Castle Street
GU1 3UQ
(01483) 504121
web@castlestudios.co.uk
www.castlestudios.co.uk

'Malcolm was very good at getting Ben to laugh and respond. We were very pleased with the reasonably priced photos.'
Cherrie, mum of Ben and James

Damian Bailey Photography
4 Lancaster Avenue
Farnham
GU9 8JY
(01252) 727351; (07971) 405152
damian@damianbailey.com
www.damianbailey.com

'We got some great photos from Damian. He was really nice and very efficient and got good reactions from the children. He comes to your house and does black and white and colour shots, some on a studio-style background and some with a more everyday background. You can get them framed or just as prints, in various sizes. He also posts them all on a personal website for a while. You choose your shots from the website and you can give the address to friends and family, to buy from or just to look at. We initially thought him quite pricey, but he isn't at all when compared to others of the same ilk.'
Tessa, mum of Daisy, Zach and Jake

Steve Wood Photography
7 Rowans Close
Farnborough
GU14 9EJ
(01276) 33054; (07919) 374531
steve@swphotography.co.uk
www.swphotography.co.uk

'Steve Wood offers the *Cherubs* photography package, whereby you take your baby to be photographed at 3-6

months, 9-12 months and 15-18 months and you then receive a free framed set of three prints. Of course, you'll no doubt buy lots of other photos that he takes at these sessions, but there is no obligation and no studio fee. In my experience the photos he takes are really lovely and not too expensive. It's a bit of a hike to Farnborough, but worth the effort and you can always combine it with a trip to the big *M&S* at Camberley!'
Julie, mum of Ben and Katie

'The deal was excellent and he has a lovely white studio, some great props and good ideas for shots, and we had some lovely memories captured.'
Michelle, mum of Annabelle

Washable Nappies

Nappies are a vital part of baby and toddler life for a few years, and if the volume and eventual fate of our rubbish troubles your conscience, washable nappies might be for you. But the vast and confusing range of possibilities can be daunting – how do washable nappies work, where do you get them and will it mean the nappy-pins and washing-lines of terry squares of my childhood? With time, space and money at a premium when you have small children, will they be worthwhile?

Fortunately the technology has moved on and here are some enthusiastic parents to guide us through it. Experimenting is easier now many suppliers and local authorities offer a trial pack – including *Guildford Borough Council* (details below). The *NCT* doesn't advocate disposables or washables but has a principle of informed choice, so here are a range of local possibilities.

Most washable nappies consist of the cloth 'nappy' part and an outer waterproof 'wrap', but there are all-in-one options too. A liner of paper or fleece catches solids and can be disposed of or washed. The *Surrey Real Nappy Network* (see p185) produces an excellent leaflet outlining the whole thing, complete with photographs of cute and comfortable babies. We have listed a selection of brands and suppliers used by local parents.

Ease of use

'Modern washable nappies are very different from the terry squares that our parents might have used. These days most washable nappies are shaped like disposables and include mod cons such as elastic round the legs, *Velcro* or poppers (not pins!) to fasten them, and an integral waterproof cover. So they're just as easy to use as disposables. Most nurseries are happy to use your washables if you provide a bag or bucket to collect the dirties in. I would also suggest that you provide any nursery with pre-assembled washables to avoid any mishaps such as

Services

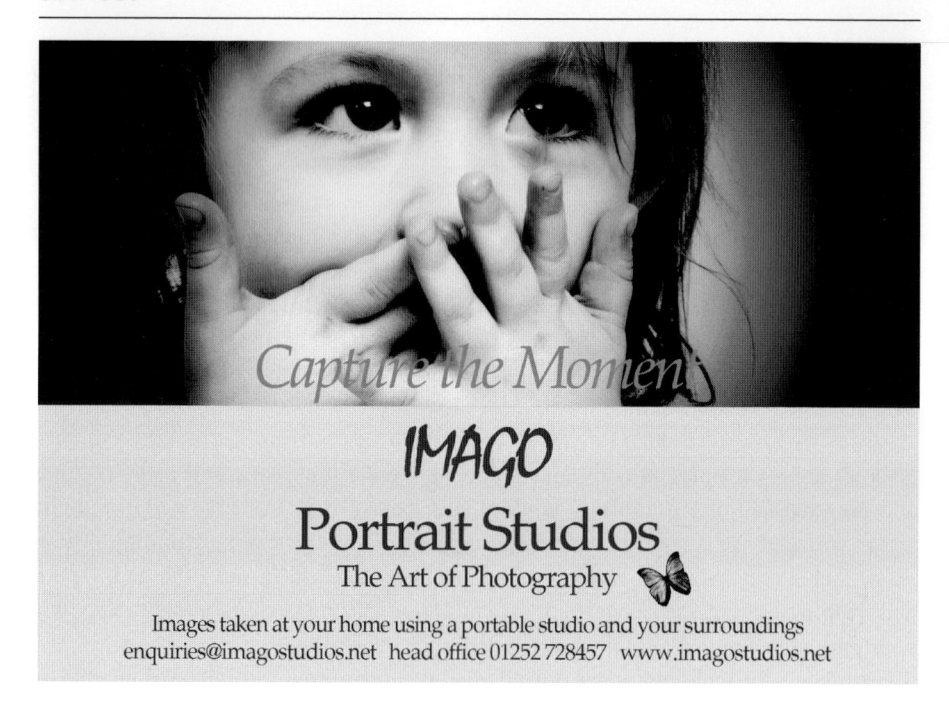

Capture the Moment
IMAGO
Portrait Studios
The Art of Photography

Images taken at your home using a portable studio and your surroundings
enquiries@imagostudios.net   head office 01252 728457   www.imagostudios.net

the omission of the poo-catching paper liner! One distinct advantage of using washables is that you don't have to keep on going shopping for heavy and bulky packs of nappies. Once you've bought them, you've got them for good, and you only really need to shop occasionally for paper liners and whatever you use to soak them in prior to washing.'
Miranda, mum of Kieron and Anthony

'We started putting Noah in washable nappies from around four months due to the disposable nappy landfill and because it works out cheaper for us than buying more and more disposable nappies. I must admit I was a bit scared in the beginning that it would be very time consuming using real nappies but I was wrong; it really is just as easy!'
Nadine and Peter, parents of Noah and Luca

Washing and drying

'We store dirty nappies in lidded buckets and then soak them in water with a few drops of tea-tree oil a couple of hours before washing them. As we have a standard washing machine, no tumble-dryer and no radiators on which to dry nappies, we opted for nappies with a separate waterproof wrap and booster pads that either open out or detach to ensure that they dry as quickly as possible on our portable clothes rack (*Tots Bots* or

Modern Baby brands suited us best). It's easy in the summer, as the rack can go outside and the nappies dry really quickly (and are softer and whiter afterwards), although not so easy in the winter.'
Miranda, mum of Kieron and Anthony

'The liners that go inside the nappy are flushable and biodegradable; so when changing Noah we just flush the liner plus poo down the toilet and we collect all the dirty nappies in a nappy bin ('dry-pailing'.) Then once the nappy bin is full we rinse them in the washing machine and then wash them either in a 40°C or 60°C wash. I tend to put a bit of *Vanish* in the wash to get rid of poo stains on the nappies. We do not use a tumble dryer but the nappies are usually dry within a day or two. We have been really happy with the *Mother-ease* nappies we bought and so far Noah has never had nappy rash.'
Nadine and Peter, parents of Noah and Luca

'I wash the nappies at 60 degrees in with the normal wash, including my husband's work shirts, and have never had any problems with this. No soaking and prewashing is required so the washing side is really much easier than I expected.

The all-in-one option takes forever to dry, so using an outer wrap and separate nappy worked much better in practice, even though it seemed like a lot of layers at first.'
Sam, mum of Freya

'We have been using washables for a year, and we have not only saved loads of money but also saved the environment! Freya never has nappy rash or chafe marks where disposables rub on the leg. They are easy to use, easy to wash and dry and the only smell is when I put the wet nappies into the washing machine. Smells are combated by drops of tea-tree oil in the bucket and lavender oil in the softener section of the washing machine.'
Colleen, mum of Freya

Comfort

'Both of our boys have been very comfortable in their washable nappies. When on holiday we tend to use disposables, which have in fact caused more problems (such as nappy rash and leaking/exploding!) than the washables. Also, washables supposedly help with potty-training because the child is more aware of being wet/dirty. I would certainly go along with this theory, given that our eldest son took only three days to be fully potty-trained (day and night!)'
Miranda, mum of Kieron and Anthony

Sources

Washable nappies are gradually becoming easier to buy off the shelf, but because of all the many possibilities available, it can be invaluable to have someone to guide you

Services

through when you start. There are a number of websites and agents who carry a variety of brands, will talk you through the options, show you the nappies and sell you the most suitable. Guildford NCT holds an introductory evening periodically for anyone thinking of using washables, where you can get a realistic view from parents who have used them (see 'All about the NCT' for details of these 'New to...' events).

'When I started investigating using washables four years ago, I had no idea just how bewildering the world of nappies could be. I had never changed a nappy before, so was struggling to assess the various merits of the numerous nappy options on the market. Also, every source of information seemed to use slightly different terminology, which added to the confusion.

Things have improved significantly since then, and the internet is a great place to find out all the information you want. However, I found it impossible to assess the nappy options without actually touching/feeling them e.g. to compare size, weight, texture, absorbency, etc., so I tapped into a network of people who sold nappies from their homes.' [Such as the ones that follow...]

Miranda, mum of Kieron and Anthony

The Nappy Lady
15 The Stanley Centre
Kelvin Way
Crawley
RH10 9SE
(0845) 6526532
www.thenappylady.co.uk

'I ordered my *Tots Bots Fluffles* from www.nappylady.co.uk. The service was excellent and my personal 'nappy lady' extremely helpful in advising me as to which nappies would suit us the best.
Colleen, mum of Freya

'We've used *Mother-ease* nappies with both children and highly recommend them. They are brilliantly designed with rows of poppers so you can adjust the size to fit babies from about 8lb up to toddlers. We've used both fleece liners and flushable ones which you can just lift out and flush away (especially good once the baby is on solids and doing proper poos!) We don't bother soaking them but just have a nappy bucket to keep the dirty ones in and then do a wash (at 40 or 60 degrees) every two to three days – it really isn't a hassle, and they dry quickly outside or on radiators (we don't have a tumble dryer). The children have always seemed totally comfortable in them and we've never had any problems with nappy rash.

We got the whole kit from the *Nappy Lady* website and paid just over £200. The website is brilliant. You can fill in an online questionnaire about your needs (drying facilities, how many children you have etc.) and it provides tailored advice and suggests different types of nappies to go for. It also sells eco-disposable nappies for times when you're not using washable

ones and provides loads of useful tips and advice.'
Jo, mum of James and Daisy

'I use *www.thenappylady.com*. There's so much information on there to help you choose including good photos and details of second-hand nappies for sale. There is a consultant service too and you get a discount if you buy through your advisor. We started using washables half and half with disposables when our daughter was newborn. We started with *Tots Bots* which were great if a bit big and 'crunchy' with the *Mother-ease Rikki* wrap. That's the best wrap I have tried – I tried the *Tots Bots* wrap among others but it was plasticky and leaky too. We also used *Fluffles* – its biggest advantage being that it doesn't need to be tumble dried – you just leave the nappies on the radiator and they're dry in an hour, and lovely and soft. However, I also found that they are really big, and 'catch' on the dry skin you invariably get on your fingertips from washing your hands twenty times a day when dealing with a newborn.

When we came to buying the next size up, having tried about a dozen types, we ended up with *Tots Bots' Bamboozle*. They're brilliant: they're slimmer than the cotton ones, which helps when fitting into clothes (one of the biggest drawbacks for me actually is not the washing but that most clothes are cut for disposables). *Bamboozles* are soft on the bum and really absorbent. I use fleece liners during the day and boosters during the night. Apart from one or two newborn poo leaks – and then nothing major, we've never had a 'poo-tastrophe' with washables like we have with the disposables. Washing isn't a big deal as you're doing so much anyway, and at least we don't have bags and bags of stinking disposables around the house in summer. Doing half and half means that we feel we have the best of both worlds – when she's at the childminder or we're out and about, we use *Huggies*. At night and at home, we use *Bamboozle*. I wouldn't even think about washables though unless you have a tumble dryer (unless you're using *Fluffles*).'
Rosie, mum of Lily

The Nappy Biz
2 Angelica Road
GU2 9GY
(01483) 833640; (07920) 051921 (Louise)
enquiries@thenappybiz.co.uk (best contact)
www.thenappybiz.co.uk

'We've used washable nappies with Tom since he was nine months old. We chose *Fluffles* by *Tots Bots* with a *Mother-ease* popper-type wrap (Tom can undo the *Velcro* type). Tracy from *The Nappy Biz* showed us an incredible variety of nappies in the comfort of our living room and after trialing a few we ended up with these.

They are adjustable and therefore fit around a pot-bellied baby comfortably (fastened with that clever *Nappi Nippas* device rather than pins these days) and they are super quick-drying as we

didn't have a tumble dryer. We also use fleece washable liners. I bought a couple and then went out and bought a metre of fleece material and cut it up into generous-sized strips to catch more poo!! Both my husband and I are really pleased we've used them and now we're used to it, we don't flinch at holding a dirty liner down the toilet to rinse it before dry-pailing. I feel they're better for Tom and the environment and he gets upset if he has to wear a disposable now!'
Heather, mum of Tom

Tots Bots
(0141) 778 7486
www.totsbots.com
Nappies available direct from the manufacturer or via various websites (see above).

'Fleecy *Tots Bots* (cutely called *Fluffles*) are quick drying but make baby look like a 'butter ball' and are too big to get trousers over (although a good option if you don't have a tumble dryer). Bamboo *Tots Bots* (*Bamboozles*) have good absorbency for low bulk but take longer to dry. Bamboo is a good eco-friendly material being more sustainable than cotton.'
Sam, mum of Freya

Guildford Borough Council
(01483) 445085 Jane Alexander
www.guildford.gov.uk

Offers a subsidised trial pack containing a range of types to allow you to find the one that suits you and your baby best.

Available to residents of the borough; other boroughs have similar schemes.

Little Green Earthlets
(0845) 072 4462
www.earthlets.co.uk

Stockists of *Mother-ease* and much else as well as a big range of other baby-related items.

Mother-ease
diapers@mother-ease.com
www.mother-ease.com

A very popular brand available from *Waitrose*, direct and from a variety of websites (see above).

NCT
(0870) 122 1120
www.nctsales.co.uk

Mail-order for various well-regarded brands of washables – *Tots Bots*, *Mother-ease* and *Yummies*, and eco-disposables – *Moltex Oko* and *Bambo Nature*.

Surrey Real Nappy Network
surreyrnn@surreycc.co.uk
www.surreywaste.info/communities/ partnership/nappy/rnn
(07768) 916276 (Dawn McCarron)

Encouraging the use of washable nappies through the county with various initiatives, including a very good leaflet and discounts from certain suppliers.

Twinkle Twinkle
(0118) 969 5550
info@twinkleontheweb.co.uk
www.twinkleontheweb.co.uk

Supplies a wide variety of brands, including eco-disposables.

Eco-friendly disposables

Moltex Oko

'I had high hopes of using washables, but what with one reason or another I never quite got round to it; and anyway, once I'd discovered *Moltex* I was perfectly happy. *Moltex* is the only nappy that is unbleached, has a soft cotton-like layer next to baby's skin, and doesn't contain all those awful chemicals that irritate baby's skin. In fact, *Moltex* and *Nature* nappies (see below) were the only ones that didn't give either of my children nappy rash. (Charlotte's bottom looked burned after wearing *Pampers* or *Huggies*). I also found that *Moltex* nappies were better at keeping moisture away from their skin. My only issue was with Louis – the nappies leaked through the top overnight as he got a bit older. So I had to switch to *Nature babycare*.

Moltex nappies are degradable. The best way to do this is to compost them or put them in a wormery; however due to the quantity of nappies we got through this wasn't feasible…roll-on nappy collections from the local council! *Moltex* can be quite expensive if bought one pack at a time, and aren't that easy to find. I found the best way to buy them was in bulk – two boxes of three packs each, each pack containing about 54 nappies, for about £60.00 from *www.naturebotts.com*, (0845) 226 2186. An internet search will bring up many other websites that sell *Moltex*.'

Emma, mum of Charlotte and Louis

Nature babycare

'*Nature* nappies are oxygen-bleached, and like *Moltex* don't contain those chemicals that can harm baby's skin. They are a bit more 'crispy' than *Moltex*, but my babies never complained, and their skin was always undamaged. I can't recall any leakage issues with *Nature*, and they are apparently 70% degradable. *Nature*

Little Treasures

Domestic Cleaning & Ironing

- Regular weekly service
- Same worker each visit
- One-off spring cleans
- Ironing collection service
- Cover for holiday & sickness
- Careful selection of workers
- Fully insured

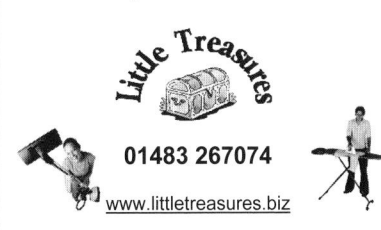

01483 267074
www.littletreasures.biz

New workers always welcome

Services

is easier to come by – the nappies are available from *Sainsbury's*, *Waitrose* and *Boots*. Now Louis is potty trained I use *Nature* pull-ups at night, and am having no problems. I buy one pack at a time as I don't know how long he'll need them for.'
Emma, mum of Charlotte and Louis

'Generally they are good; I like the fact that they are eco-friendly and I'm not filling landfill with loads of plastic – you should really also use the biodegradable nappy sacs (also made by *Nature*) or there's not much point using the nappy! I feel less guilty about not using washables, but then again, once you've taken into account all the electricity and detergent used to wash and dry them, I'm not sure how much better washables are anyway.

Nature nappies are as easy to use as any other nappy, but quite bulky. I tend to use *Huggies* at night because they leak less and keep the wee away from the skin better over long periods. I do find *Nature* slightly more expensive.'
Louise, mum of Sophie and Phoebe

Other eco-friendly disposables

Tushies, Bambo Nature, Weenees, Imse Vimse, Tendercare etc. are available direct through many websites. You will be able to find them through a basic internet search.

Information Centres

Guildford Library, the *Tourist Information Centre* and *Citizens Advice Bureau (CAB)* are all right in the centre of town. With luck, you may never need to call on the services of the *CAB*, but the *Library* is especially valuable with children and at the *Tourist Information Centre* you can keep up to date with the vast array of local events and attractions, and often book tickets on the spot. The *Mobile Library Service* and the *Toy Library* provide even more local resources.

Citizens Advice Bureau
15-21 Haydon Place
GU1 4LL
(01483) 576699 (telephone advice 10.00 am – 12.00 pm weekdays)
(01483) 506886 (appointments line)
www.guildfordcab.org.uk
Mon – Fri 10.00 am – 4.00 pm
Thurs 10.00 am – 7.00 pm
Sat 10.00 am – 12.00 pm

Appointment only – weekday afternoons and Thursday 4.00 – 7.00 pm

An advice service for everybody, staffed by trained volunteers, to 'help resolve legal, money and other problems by offering free, independent and confidential advice.' They will help you understand the system for welfare, benefits, housing and a huge variety of other areas and refer you on to the most suitable body.

Guildford Library

77 North Street
GU1 4AL
(08456) 009009
libraries@surreycc.gov.uk
www.surreycc.gov.uk
Mon, Fri and Sat 9.30 am – 8.00 pm
Tues and Thurs 9.30 am – 5.00 pm
Wednesday 9.30 am – 1.00 pm
Thursday 9.30 am – 5.00 pm

Children's Library

'The Children's Space @ Guildford Library is exactly that – a space for children and their accompanying adults to relax, read, chat and even use the computers. It is colourful, fun and completely aimed at young children. There are bags of board books for babies, picture books for toddlers and older children, easy-to-read books and children's stories (although there is no subscription to any reading schemes such as the *Oxford Reading Tree*), and lots of non-fiction for all ages. If there's a book you want but it's not at Guildford you can order it in from another library.

CD-ROMs are available for hire, as are music CDs, story tapes, videos and DVDs. There are also books to help children with a particular situation, such as divorce, gaining a sibling, death, going to the dentist, etc. There are computers available for use with CD-ROM facilities and internet access, and printing is also available. There are also study tables set aside for older children.

Unfortunately there is not a dedicated children's librarian and there are times when the desk is not staffed but assistance can normally be found. All staff are very keen and knowledgeable.

On Friday there is a story time for preschool children, and on Tuesday there is a very popular '*Baby Bounce and Rhyme*' session [see full review on p46 *Things to do*]. During the year there are special events such as a visiting story teller, illustrator or an Easter egg hunt. There are also events for *National Children's Book Week* and the *Guildford Book Festival*.

The library participates in two national schemes for encouraging reading.

ABACUS
Baby & Party Hire

For Hire of good quality
Baby & Nursery Equipment

Cots* travel cots*highchairs*car seats*buggies
incl. All Terrain*Z beds*musical baby swings etc.

AND FOR PARTIES
Small tables & chairs*slide*tunnels*ballpond
*roller coaster*pop-up castles

AND FOR GARDEN PARTIES
Patio tables*chairs*parasols*
gazebos*party tents

FOR MORE DETAILS AND PRICES
Telephone ELIZABETH on 01483 285142
www.babyhire.co.uk

Services

Bookstart is for babies and young children, inviting them to join the library and providing them with free books. When your baby has six stamps for visiting the library, he gets another *Bookstart* bag. The *National Summer Reading Scheme* encourages children to read a certain number of books over the summer holidays for which they receive stickers and pencils etc., and are presented with an award at the end.

Children who join the library now get a colourful Maisy card and are not charged fines.

Adult library

'For grown-ups there are books, videos, DVDs, music CDs, talking tapes, newspapers and a reference section. There are computers with free internet access, word processing, printing and access to the online reference service.

Enquiries Direct

c/o Guildford Library (address above)
(01483) 543599
libraries@surreycc.gov.uk
www.surreycc.gov.uk [click on learning, libraries, information services, enquiries direct]

'There is no longer an Information Centre in Guildford library but you can ring or email any enquiry to Enquiries Direct and the staff there will get back to you as soon as they can.'
Jane Cook, former librarian and mum of Josh and Isobel

Urban Mobile Library Service

(01483) 517402 (call for exact locations and times of stops)
www.surreycc.gov.uk (detailed timetable)

Monday: Burpham/Stoughton/ Goldsworth Park
Tuesday: Merrow Street and Bushy Hill/ Onslow Village/Worplesdon
Wednesday: Windlesham
Thursday: Goldsworth Park/Park Barn/ Stoughton
Friday: Dennisville/Shalford/Shere/ Westborough
Saturday: Frimley/Heatherside

'Library has a small but interesting children's section. Children just love climbing up on the bus and sitting on the little seat to look at the books. Very friendly staff too.'
Helen, mum of Dominic and Laura

Godalming Toy Library

Broadwater Park Community Centre
Summers Road
GU7 3BH
(01483) 424307 (Kirsten)
Tuesday (inc holidays) 2.00 – 4.00 pm
www.surreycc.gov.uk

'Friendly atmosphere where you are welcome to hire toys for two weeks at reasonable prices or just come and play.

Toys are geared towards preschool children but all ages are welcome. There is a spacious hall with lots of exciting toys for children to play with and hire. There's plenty of room to try out a wide range of toys including large outdoor toys. An ideal place to go, especially in bad weather. Plenty of free parking available adjacent to hall.

It is located next to Broadwater Park [see *Places to Visit* p107], which has a lovely children's play area and ducks to feed.'

Cathy, mum of Hannah

The Tourist Information Centre
14 Tunsgate
GU1 3QT
(01483) 444333
www.guildford.gov.uk

May – September:
Monday – Saturday 9.00 am – 5.30 pm;
Sunday 10.00 am – 4.30 pm
October – April:
Monday – Saturday 9.30 am – 5.00 pm

An excellent source of information on local events and entertainment, places to visit, how to get there and where to stay. You can book accommodation, buy tickets for many local events, and buy guidebooks, maps, and so forth. There is in-depth coverage for local events and information, but information is also available for the rest of the country.

8

Health and Welfare

Dimitra Stamogiannou, mum of Electra
Maggie Sherborne, mum of Alice and Katy

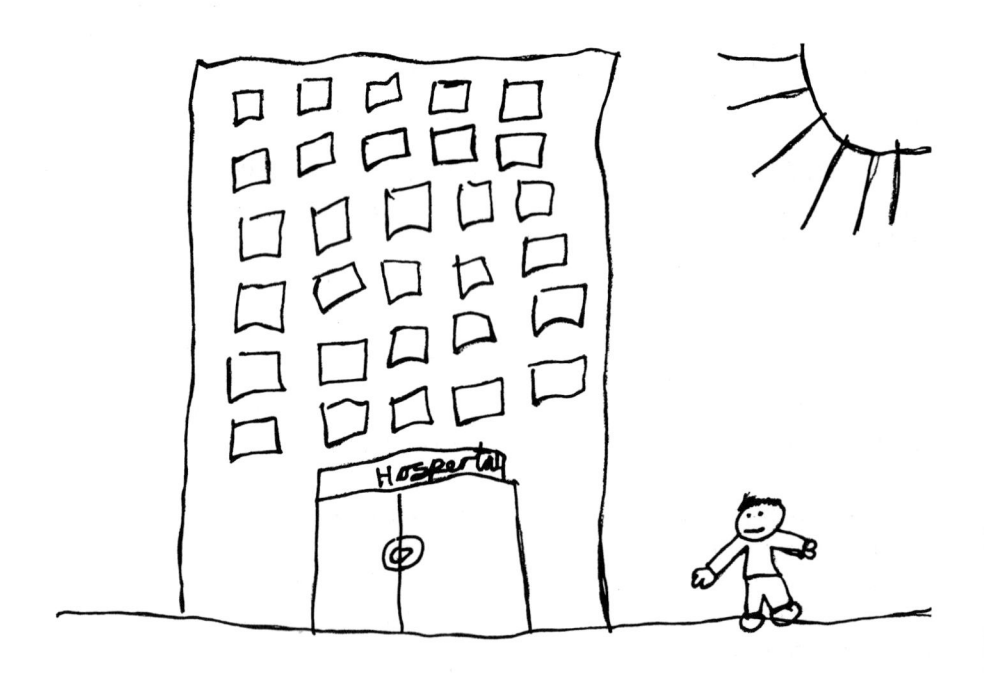

The health and wellbeing of your little ones as well as your own always raises many questions. What medical services are available? Where can I find a dentist? What do I do if my child needs glasses? Who should I turn to if I need breastfeeding support and advice?

This section provides an overview of the services and support networks that are available to you and offers some practical advice and information.

Health and Welfare

Healthcare Provision

GP Surgeries

When you first move into an area, it is very important to find your local GP surgery and to register your whole family. Do not leave it until you are ill because many surgeries will not give you an appointment unless you are already registered with them (although they might do as a one-off). Most GP practices have a catchment area and are usually unwilling to take patients from outside that area. Unless you have a definite reason for registering elsewhere, it is normally a good idea to use your local surgery so that you can get there as easily as possible in an emergency.

Austen Road Surgery
1 Austen Road, GU1 3NW
(01483) 564578
www.austenroadsurgery.co.uk

Dapdune Surgery
Dapdune House, Wharf Road,
Woodbridge Road, GU1 4RP
(0844) 4778900

East Horsley Medical Centre
Kingston Avenue, East Horsley,
Leatherhead, KT24 6QT
(01483) 284151
www.horsleydocs.co.uk

Fairlands Practice
Fairlands Medical Centre, Fairlands
Avenue, Worplesdon, GU3 3NA
(01483) 594250
www.fairlands.co.uk
Normandy Branch Surgery, Glaziers Lane,
Normandy, GU3 2DD
(01483) 813274
www.fairlands.co.uk

Guildowns Group Practice
The Surgery, 91/93 Wodeland Avenue,
GU2 4YP
The Oaks Surgery, Applegarth Avenue,
Park Barn, GU2 8LZ
Stoughton Road Surgery, 2 Stoughton
Road, GU1 1LL
The Student Heath Centre, Stag Hill,
University of Surrey, GU2 7HX
(0844) 477 3051
www.guildowns.nhs.uk

Merrow Park Surgery
Kingfisher Drive, Merrow, GU4 7EP
(01483) 503331

New Inn Surgery
202 London Road, Burpham, GU4 7JS
(01483) 301091
www.newinnsurgery.co.uk

Peaslake Surgery
Peaslake Lane, Peaslake, GU5 9R
(01306) 730875

Health and Welfare

Shere Surgery
Gomshall Lane, Shere, GU5 9DR
(01483) 202066
www.sheremedicalcentre.co.uk

St Luke's Surgery
Warren Road, GU1 3JH
(0844) 4778716
www.stlukes.gpsurgery.net/Webdesk/
netblast/pages/index.html

St Nicolas Surgery
Buryfields, GU2 4AZ
(01483) 303200

Villages Medical Centre
Send Barns Lane, Send, Woking, GU23 7BP
(01483) 226330
www.thevillagesmc.co.uk

Wonersh Surgery
The Street, Wonersh, GU5 0PE
(01483) 898123
www.wonershsurgery.org.uk

Woodbridge Hill Surgery
1 Deerbarn Road, GU2 8YB
(0844) 4778663
www.woodbridgehillsurgery.co.uk

See also – www.gawcrd.org.uk/gp_directory.htm – for a complete list of doctors and surgeries further afield in Surrey.

Health Visitors

All surgeries have a health visitor linked to them. Health visitors usually run a weekly baby clinic at the surgery to weigh babies and to answer any questions that concerned parents may have. There is often a nurse at these clinics to give immunisations and a doctor who will see the children when necessary. These clinics do not offer appointments; you are simply seen in order of arrival. It can sometimes be a long wait so use it as an opportunity to meet other local mums! Different surgeries hold baby clinics on different days. If you cannot attend the baby clinic at your surgery, you can attend the clinic at a different surgery as long as you have your child's red *'Personal Child Health Record'* book.

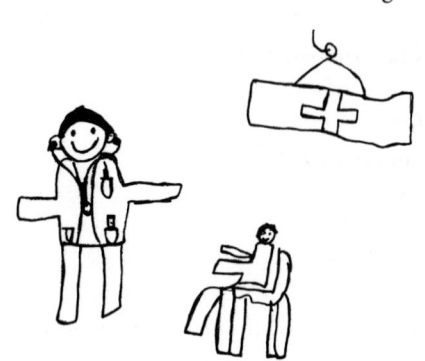

In addition to weekly clinics, health visitors arrange postnatal classes for mums with young babies – also excellent ways of meeting other new mums in your area. Remember that your health visitor is there to help you as a parent. If you have any concerns about your child's

Health and Welfare

```
            Emma Hobbs
          Raw Dip and ITEC

          Holistic Health
         & Beauty Therapist

Dermalogica, Jessica & Fake Bake Products used

Beauty Treatments Including:
Facials        Manicures & Pedicures
Massage        Tanning              Waxing
Weddings       Eye Lash Tinting     Pamper Parties
                                    Eye Brow Tinting

Gift Vouchers Available

Call For An Appointment: 07779 269214
```

development, whether it be feeding, sleeping, physical development or behaviour, then speak to a health visitor. If they are not in when you ring, do leave a message. Your local surgery will be able to give you the contact number for your health visitor.

Each surgery also has a community midwife linked to it. For straightforward pregnancies this midwife and her team will be your main carers antenatally and postnatally. They will do your check-ups at their weekly clinic at the surgery, and will arrange your scans at the hospital. For the first 10 days after the birth of your baby the midwives will visit you at home. After this the health visitor becomes your main contact.

Accident and Emergency (A&E)
Royal Surrey County Hospital
Egerton Road
GU2 7XX
(01483) 571122
webfeedback@royalsurrey.nhs.uk
www.royalsurrey.nhs.uk

For injuries and illnesses that can't wait for an appointment, or if you haven't got around to registering with a practice yet and you need to see a doctor, you can go to Accident and Emergency at the *Royal Surrey County Hospital* (*RSCH*) (beyond *Tesco*, just off the A3 at the cathedral exit). You will initially be assessed by a nurse and then referred on to a doctor if necessary. It might involve rather a long wait.

Thamesdoc (out-of-hours GP services)
(0208) 3909991
www.thamesdoc.org

NHS Direct
(0845) 4647
www.nhsdirect.nhs.uk

For information and advice about health, illness and health services, you can also call *NHS Direct*, which provides a 24-hour telephone health line, and e-health information services to the public.

Alternative Therapies

[See also p54 under *Things to do* for baby massage and yoga for babies and adults, and reflexology]

Chiropractor
Back to Health
5 Jenner Road
GU1 3PH
(01483) 306 538

'I started going to the chiropractor when my eldest daughter was 18 months old as

Health and Welfare

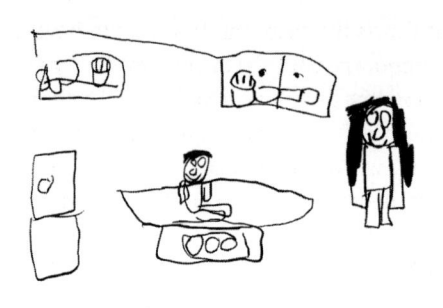

my back had never really recovered from giving birth. In only a couple of weeks of fairly intensive appointments I found that I was sleeping better and felt much stronger. I continued going throughout my second pregnancy and since the birth of my second daughter, and it has been of great help with all the aches and pains that are caused by carrying heavy children. The staff are really friendly and I have always felt completely at ease. There is a box of toys and crayons to keep little ones occupied and they are all very good at looking after a screaming baby! They also offer chiropractic care to children.'
Katherine, mum of Holly and Hazel

Cranial Osteopath – Ann Cook
8 Upper Guildown Road
GU2 4EZ
(01483) 504508

'I have taken both my children to see Ann and have been amazed at how much she has been able to help them with cranial osteopathy. My son suffered from terrible colic and was treated from when he was eight weeks old. At the first appointment, Ann takes a full history of everything that may be relevant to the treatment she will give, ranging from pregnancy ailments, labour, birth and post-birth. The treatment itself is very gentle, lasts about half an hour and babies seem to enjoy it – I could see my son visibly relax during his treatment. After four sessions his colic was hugely improved. I'm currently taking my daughter to see Ann after a traumatic birth and subsequent inability to settle at night and after one session I've seen an improvement. Cranial osteopathy isn't a cure-all, but if you are having problems with your baby, it's definitely worth giving an osteopath a call.'
Julie, mum of Ben and Katie

Cranial Osteopath – Chris Grey
Wishing Well
52A College Street
Petersfield
GU31 4AF
(01730) 233802

The Holistic Centre
Wiggins Yard
Bridge Street
Godalming
GU7 1HW
(01483) 418103

'I took both my tiny babies to see a cranial osteopath after he'd been hailed by many of my friends as 'God'. Cranial osteopathy looks odd – it's a very gentle manipulation of the skull and the rest of the body and helps to eliminate the traumas of birth and to ensure all 'channels' are free-flowing. Charlotte and Louis both had terrible all-day-long colic, which vanished after a few sessions. I could see then visibly relax during the sessions, they always slept better afterwards, and in fact, Charlotte bestowed her first smile, during one of her sessions, on the osteopath (traitor!)

I've seen him reverse sleep patterns on babies that were asleep all day and awake all night, and he has helped to relieve Louis' chest where he has a tendency to infections. Some say it's witchcraft – I don't care, it's harmless and it works. And when you've been pacing the tiles night after night, it's worth it!'

Emma, mum of Charlotte and Louis

Finding a Dentist

Taking your child

'It is never too early to take your child to the dentist. If you have a dentist you see regularly take your children along with you and find out what they do for kids and how often they will want to do check ups. If you do not have a dentist, now is the time to get one. NHS dentistry is free during pregnancy and until your child is one year old.

During pregnancy

'You can have a full range of treatments while you are pregnant. This includes dental X-rays, although do note that the dentist is X-raying your teeth not your baby, and the dose of radiation to you is less than you would get on a flight to Spain. The only treatment dentists avoid is amalgam fillings and a certain local anaesthetic injection which is rarely used anyway.

White fillings are not always possible especially if the filling is really close to or going under your gingiva (gums), so if this is the case you may have to have a temporary filling until you have had your baby. The best time to have treatment is in the middle trimester, so get your check-up early in your pregnancy so you can have any necessary treatment done before you get large and uncomfortable. Even if your baby is over a year old remember NHS dentistry is cheap. It costs about £17.00 just for a check up, X-rays and scaling, about £45.00 for fillings and extractions (for the entire course of treatment, not per filling), and about £200.00 if you need any crowns or bridges.

The NHS will not pay for cosmetic treatment, for example, tooth whitening, large white fillings or white crowns on back teeth. You can opt to have these provided privately.

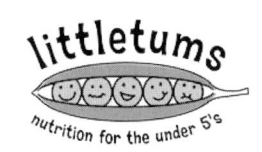

---

littletums

nutrition for the under 5's

**Thinking about weaning?
Frustrated with a fussy eater?
Or just wanting to optimise your child's diet?**

Why not see if I can help?

Book an evening talk for you & your friends;

**'Weaning and the Weaning Diet'
'Healthy Eating for the Under 5's'
'Managing Fussy Eaters'**

or an individual consultation to discuss your child's diet in detail

**Lucy Schneiderman BSc Hons.
Registered Nutritionist
07941 992 355
lucy@littletums.co.uk
www.littletums.co.uk**

Health and Welfare

Dental Care for Children

Dr Sarah Lyle BDS LDS DDPH RCS(Eng)
Specialist in Children's Dentistry

Sarah has been practising children's dentistry for over 25 years and believes that a healthy mouth helps a child to smile, eat and talk with confidence.

Children can reach adulthood well-educated in oral care, free from active disease and relaxed about visiting the dentist.

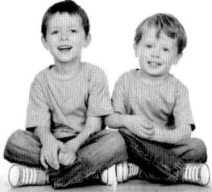

RINGLEY PARK Dental Practice
59 Reigate Road Reigate Surrey RH2 0QZ
Tel: 01737 240123
Fax: 01737 245704
Email: info@ringleypark.org
Web: www.ringleypark.org

Finding an NHS Dentist

(0845) 271 2040 *(if you live in Surrey)*
(0845) 0508345 *(if you live in Hampshire)*
These numbers also work if you have a dental emergency.

'Alternatively, you can look on the web at *www.nhs.uk*. A search facility allows you to enter your postcode and will list local dentists and what NHS services (if any) each practice provides.'
Maggie Sherborne, senior dental officer and mum of Alice and Katy

If your child needs glasses or has eye problems

Go and see your doctor initially if your child is too young to go to a high street optician. If your GP thinks it is necessary you will be referred to a specialist at the hospital. The *RSCH* has a dispensing optician where prescriptions are made and filled. However, this is only available on Wednesdays, so if the glasses need repairing or replacing, you will need to wait a week.

'My daughter, Alice, was 15 months old when given her first pair. With a neighbour's help and by feeding her a banana, we tied the glasses onto her, but she had them off and broken beyond repair within 24 hours. The second pair lasted three days. It improved from then on but for the first eight months or so the average life of a pair of specs was three weeks before they either needed replacing or repairing. I rang the hospital when she broke the first pair (on a Thursday) and was informed that I could not take them in until the following Wednesday. I would then get the glasses back the Wednesday after that. Unfortunately, the shop that supplied the hospital did not stock small children's frames outside the hospital.

When your child's glasses get broken, you have to go back to the shop that gave you the original prescription to get the free NHS replacement or repair. Therefore my advice is, when you are given your initial prescription go somewhere on the high street that does fast in-shop lenses so you do not have to wait long. We are now regular visitors to *Vision Express* on Guildford High Street. I have found the staff to be always helpful, and the store usually has a choice of frames for Alice to choose from. We go in with the broken pair, choose the replacement, then retreat to a café or to see ducks for an hour while the glasses are made up. Alice is now nearly three and has had her current pair six months.

My neighbour also has a tot in glasses and has reported that she has found *Specsavers* helpful with a good range of frames to choose from.'

Maggie, mum of Alice and Katy

Breastfeeding

NCT Breastfeeding Counsellors

(0870) 444 8708 – NCT National Breastfeeding Line manned daily 8.00 am – 10.00 pm
www.nctpregnancyandbabycare.com

The *NCT* actively promotes breastfeeding because of its many advantages to both mother and baby, and offers support to all parents however they decide to feed their baby. Breastfeeding counsellors offer free and confidential information and advice.

The *NCT* breastfeeding counsellor serving the Guildford area is Alison Taylor who can be contacted on (01483) 857595.

Guildford Drop-In Breastfeeding Clinic

Wednesday 10.30 – 12.30

Held in the parentcraft room at the *RSCH*, this clinic is open to anybody with a baby or child who would like one-to-one support on all aspects of breastfeeding.

La Leche League of Guildford

(0845) 120 2918 (for breastfeeding help)
LLLguildford@tye-walker.co.uk (for details of local get-togethers)
www.laleche.org.uk

La Leche League (LLL) is the leading international breastfeeding support organisation and there are groups all over the world providing mother-to-mother support and information.

LLL of Guildford is a friendly and lively group that meets on a regular basis. Meetings are like coffee mornings, with a theme, during which experiences are shared about breastfeeding and mothering. Topics include beginning breastfeeding, overcoming challenges, first foods for the breastfed baby and

---

MAKE SENSE OF IT ALL

Private and confidential Counselling/Therapy available

Louise Campbell

Ad.Dip Integrative Humanistic Counselling
NCT A/N Teacher, Health Visitor, District Nurse

♦ Qualified therapist and Member of BACP

I am experienced in ante-natal and post-natal issues, birth experiences and depression, as well as general life difficulties.

- Free initial consultation
- Burpham area (easy parking)

Please call 07833 568058 for an informal chat or email louise@campbell.uk.com

Health and Welfare

nursing older babies and toddlers. You can also borrow books from the library.

All *LLL* leaders are accredited breastfeeding counsellors.

The Association of Breastfeeding Mothers
(0870) 401 7711 (24-hour counselling helpline)
www.abm.me.uk

This is a charity that provides information and support on all aspects of breastfeeding. The *ABM* counsellors are themselves mothers who have enjoyed breastfeeding their own babies.

The Breastfeeding Network
(0870) 900 8787 (support line operates 9.30 am – 9.30 pm daily)
www.breastfeedingnetwork.org.uk

The Breastfeeding Network staff are volunteers who have undergone extensive training and are mothers who have breastfed their babies.

9
Childcare

Katherine Thompson, mum of Holly and Hazel

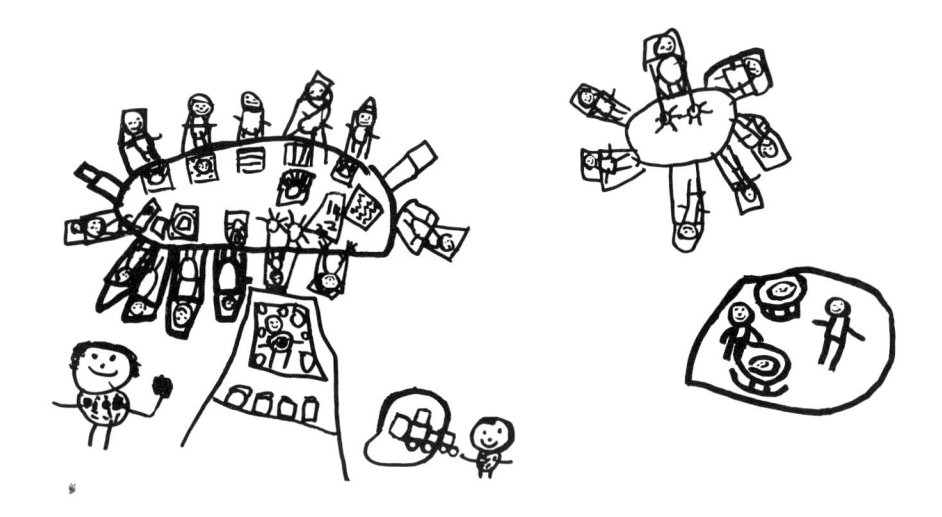

All families come up against the knotty problem of childcare at some point, whether or not both parents are working. There are so many factors to consider when choosing the childcare that will suit your circumstances best – budget, organisational requirements, the environment you would like for your child, what is available to you – that every decision is unique. In this chapter we hope to give you an outline of the choices available and some useful starting places for your research.

Childcare in Guildford is in huge demand so start looking as early as possible and try to be prepared to be flexible as to your hours if you are hoping to work part-time.

Please note that while the information in this chapter is correct as at the time of print, legislation does change and therefore we suggest that you use the contact details given through the chapter to check for any changes. In addition, an advertisement of a relevant business in this section does not constitute a recommendation.

Daycare Nurseries

Daycare nurseries vary in size, opening hours, and the ages of children that they will take; however, most will accept babies from three or four months old up until the age that they start school. Most are open from 8.00 am to 6.00 pm, and although some nurseries will take children earlier and later, there will be an additional fee for this. In addition, they often offer morning or afternoon sessions if you do not need childcare for the whole day, but the cost of this may be two-thirds of a whole day's fee.

All nurseries tend to be oversubscribed, and in some cases will take a baby's name before it is born, so it is worth putting your name on a waiting list as early as possible. That said, if for one reason or another you haven't done so, don't despair, it is still worth making the rounds in case places aren't taken up.

Daycare nurseries that follow the *National Curriculum*'s foundation stage for three to five-year-olds should be able to claim the *Nursery Education Grant* for free part-time early education. In addition, some nurseries will accept the *Childcare Voucher Scheme* [see more information under 'Paying For It' later in this chapter]. You should check with the nursery whether it subscribes to either or both schemes.

Ofsted (*Office for Standards in Education*) regulates daycare nurseries, and imposes regular inspections to ensure standards of staffing, safety and provision. *Ofsted* reports are available from *www.ofsted.gov.uk*.

A full list of daycare nurseries in the area can be found on the *Surrey County Council*'s Children's Information Service at *www.childcarelink.gov.uk* or on (08456) 011777.

The *National Day Nurseries Association* – (0870) 774 4244 – and *Sure Start* – *www.surestart.gov.uk* – have useful information and guidance on choosing a day nursery.

Below is a list of things to think about when looking at a daycare nursery – it is not exhaustive, but will give you some pointers to the sort of things to ask and look out for:

- Your gut feeling – what one parent feels is right for their child may not be what you feel is right for you and yours.
- Recommendations from friends.
- The Ofsted report.
- What is the routine? Nurseries have a routine that may be different to yours.
- Cleanliness – does the place look clean even in the midst of 'baked bean play' and potty-training children having accidents?
- What is the attitude to potty training?
- Are carers prepared to use reusable nappies?
- Will carers change children as soon as they notice they are dirty, or do they wait until 'nappy changing time'?
- Do the children look calm, safe and happy?

- Are there plenty of clean toys for the children to use?
- Is there an outdoor play area? How often do the children get outdoors?
- What are the sleeping arrangements?
- Do the carers appear to enjoy their work and being with children?
- What food is provided? Can staff provide you with a sample menu?
- What examples of the children's artwork are around the nursery?
- Are the children playing well together?
- How will you find out what your child has done all day? Some nurseries provide a 'day sheet', some provide feedback on a weekly or monthly basis.

Preschools

While children start school in the academic year that they turn five, many parents like their child to attend a preschool from the age of two-and-a-half to three, to prepare them for school. Preschools have a range of titles, including playgroups, playschools, nursery schools and *Montessori* nurseries. Some schools (both state and private) have an affiliated preschool, and it is worth checking with local infant and junior schools to see if that is the case, particularly if there is a school that you would like your child to attend.

Whichever preschool you choose, they all aim to develop the learning and social skills children will need for school. The *Government's National Curriculum – foundation stage* – aims for children to achieve certain early-learning goals by the end of the reception year, mostly through structured play. Most preschools will follow this curriculum. You can find more detailed information about the foundation stage at *www.direct.gov.uk/en/EducationAndLearning*.

Preschools usually offer either morning or afternoon sessions that last two-and-a-half to three hours. Children usually attend one session a day commonly starting with only one or two sessions a week and building up to four or five as they get closer to starting infant school.

There are two state preschools in Guildford (in addition to the state primary schools with attached nursery classes). These are The Children's Centre (town centre site), York Road, (01483) 561652 and The Children's Centre (North Guildford site), Hazel Avenue, (01483) 566589 [See p14, 18 and 64 *Things to do* for Play and Learn reviews]. They accept children from three years old, and are free from the moment they start. All other preschools, however, charge fees and you should expect to pay £7.00–£10.00 per session. Payments are made at the beginning of each half term.

All children are entitled to a government-funded foundation stage place from the term after the child turns three; this could be at a preschool, the Children's Centre, or even with some accredited childminders. However not all preschools or playgroups claim the *Nursery Education Grant*, and due to oversubscription at those preschools that do, it may not always be possible to benefit from such a place. Even if the preschool does receive this grant you may need to pay a small top-up fee if the sessions last longer than two-and-a-half hours. The preschool will claim the grant for your child at the appropriate time so you will not need to worry about making any applications.

Any preschool that opens for more than two hours a day must be registered with *Ofsted*, and is regularly inspected to ensure standards of staffing, safety and provision. *Ofsted* reports are available from *www.ofsted.gov.uk*.

A full list of preschools in the area can be found on the *Surrey County Council Children's Information Service* at *www.childcarelink.gov.uk*, or (08456) 011777.

Sure Start (*www.surestart.gov.uk*) has useful information and guidance on choosing a preschool including a list of questions to ask.

The website *www.under5s.co.uk* has useful information and links relating to education for the under-fives.

The questions in the above list of things to think about when looking at a daycare nursery all still apply when looking for a preschool. In addition you might like to ask:

- How is the preschool funded and does it receive the Nursery Education Grant?
- Is the place clean, even with all the messy activities taking place?
- What is the toilet policy? Do children have to ask to go? Or can they go at will? Do carers ensure that the children wash their hands afterwards?
- What snacks are provided?
- What are the procedures for monitoring and reporting on a child's behaviour?
- How are the children grouped and how many of them are in a class?
- How much input do parents have on what is taught?

Childminders

Childminders are self-employed and look after children in their own homes. They must be registered with *Ofsted* if they are paid to look after children up to eight years old for more than two hours a day in their home. This means that they are inspected regularly to ensure that the care they provide meets the national standards for under eight-year-olds, that their homes are suitable and that they and all adults in the house have satisfactory criminal record checks.

Childminders set their own hours and therefore might be able to offer greater flexibility to suit your circumstances and fit in with other childcare that you may have, for instance dropping off and picking up your child from preschool. They can also take your child to playgroups, to the park and on other outings. Childminders can look after more than one child; the maximum number of children of different ages that they can be in charge of is set out on their registration certificate, and you should ask to see this. Obviously as the childminder will be the sole adult carer for your child, the choice of childminder is very personal and you should make sure that you, and your child, are happy with your choice. You should enter into a contract with your childminder that will set out the terms of your agreement as to hours, fees, and arrangements for holidays and sickness.

The *Surrey County Council Children's Service* has a list of all registered childminders, and has some suggested questions that parents can ask, at *www.childcarelink.gov.uk*. In addition, speak to your friends who may be able to give recommendations. *Sure Start* also has a booklet – '*Looking for childcare*' at *www.surestart.gov.uk*.

Below is a list of things to think about when looking at childminders – it is not exhaustive, but will give you some pointers of the sort of things to ask and look out for:

- Can you see the childminder's registration certificate?
- Can you see a current public liability insurance certificate?
- How does the childminder relate to the children?
- Can you have the phone numbers of other parents that the childminder works for so you can follow up references?
- Does the childminder have an emergency arrangement with another childminder?
- Can the childminder show you around his/her home and tell you about hygiene and safety?
- Are pets managed safely?
- Does the childminder or any other adult in the house smoke?
- Check that all the rooms and the garden are insured, otherwise your child will be excluded from those areas.
- What food will be provided?
- What is the approach to toilet training?
- How does he/she spend the day and how do the other children's schedules fit in with your child?
- Who supplies milk, nappies, babyfood etc.?
- Does the childminder claim the *Nursery Education Grant*?

Crèches

A crèche can provide occasional care, full daycare or morning/afternoon care for children under eight years old at particular premises. If it is open for more than two hours a day and more than five days a week then it must be registered with *Ofsted* and therefore regularly inspected to ensure standards are maintained.

Some crèches are set up on a permanent basis, often at gyms and in shopping centres. Often crèches will be set up temporarily for a specific event to look after children while their parents are attending that event.

Fees will vary but you can expect to pay £2.00–£5.00 for a few hours care, and you usually pay per session. Some crèches (for instance at the *Spectrum*) can be very busy and often require pre-booking.

A list of registered crèches is available at *www.childcarelink.gov.uk*.

Nannies

Nannies are employed by you to look after your child in your home. Like childminders, they may be able to provide greater flexibility for your childcare arrangements. However, unlike childminders, they are not required to be registered with *Ofsted*, and it is up to you to make sure that you are happy with the person you employ.

There are various considerations to take into account when you are thinking of employing a nanny. Unlike other forms of childcare, you become an employer with various legal duties and responsibilities such as paying the Income Tax and National Insurance for your nanny. In addition, you will be responsible for safety in your home, not only for your child, but also for the nanny.

There are no legal limits on the number, or age of children that a nanny can look after; so if you have more than one child requiring daycare, this option could be cheaper than a full-time place at a day nursery. In addition, it might be possible to find a nanny share where two families jointly employ a nanny to look after their children, either together or on different days of the week.

Most people find their nannies through an agency. Agencies will carry out some of their own checks on nannies, but you should check these carefully, and also any references. An agency may be able to help with some of the legal paperwork required in employing a nanny. Nannies can also be found by word of mouth or through local advertising.

Although nannies are not required to be registered they can voluntarily choose to be put on the *Ofsted Childcare Register* – *www.ofsted.gov.uk,* (08456) 404040 – which has been open for registration since April 2007. For a fee to cover checks, nannies can be approved for 12 months at a time. The benefit to parents is some reassurance that the nanny has a minimum level of qualifications and first-aid training, and that criminal checks have been carried out. Additionally, parents employing an 'approved' nanny can qualify for help through *Working Tax Credits* and the *Employer Voucher Schemes* detailed in the section 'Paying for it' below.

There are a few general things you should decide before advertising for a nanny; here is a non-exhaustive list of some of the matters that you should consider:

- What duties do you expect your nanny to carry out?
- What hours do you want your nanny to work?
- Do you want the nanny to live in, or come on a daily basis?
- Do you have any special requirements, for instance a nanny with a second language?
- Will you be happy with a nanny who smokes?
- Do you want the nanny to be able to drive?
- How much do you want to pay and what is your budget for activities?

Obviously, the choice of nanny is a very personal matter, however when interviewing potential nannies there are a number of items that you should ask for. Again the list below is not exhaustive:

- Is the nanny on the *Ofsted Childcare Register* or *Childcare Approval Scheme*, and can he/she provide you with the approval certificate?
- Can you see two forms of identity, such as passport and driving licence?
- Can the nanny provide two referees and a full employment history?
- Would the nanny be prepared to get a GP's letter confirming his/her physical fitness to look after children?
- Can you see the nanny's qualification certificates?

Sure Start (www.surestart.gov.uk) also has tips for interviewing and questions to ask.

Au pairs

Au pairs are usually young women from abroad who are staying in the country for a limited period, either as part of their studies of the language, or for the experience. They live with the family and in return for board, food and a small wage they help with childcare and domestic tasks. The amount that au pairs are expected to do, and the responsibility they are given, varies enormously, but they would usually have some time off each day for their studies. Most au pairs do not come with childcare qualifications and would stay for three to 12 months. People often arrange au pairs through family and friends, but there are several au pair agencies in the Guildford area specialising in au pairs from different parts of the world. Like nannies, au pairs can voluntarily register with the *Ofsted Childcare Register*.

Mother's Help

Mother's Helps are employed to help around the house in whatever way is needed. They will do childcare, cooking, cleaning, laundry and shopping as well as being a companion for the mother. They are often employed for the first few months after a baby is born in order to look after the house so that Mum can concentrate on looking after the new baby. Their qualifications vary but many simply come with the experience of having been a mum themselves. Most people find mother's helps by going through an agency, but remember to check references carefully.

Babysitting

Finding a reliable babysitter is often difficult when you do not have family nearby or you are new to the area. There are one or two babysitting agencies that cover the Guildford area. Using an agency is often an expensive option; however overall, you get extremely competent babysitters with childcare experience who can do as many hours as you need. If you really want to go out to something special then these services are extremely useful.

There are also many small babysitting circles in existence. Most of these are simply groups of friends who have organised a system where tokens are exchanged for babysitting. The most successful circles have 10-15 members who all know each other and are fairly local to one another. To find out about these groups you just need to ask around, or failing that, you could start up one of your own. Mention it to two or three friends and get them to mention it to some of their friends. Have a few socials so that everyone can get to know each other. Sort out a token or points system, then have lots of nights out! And there you have it, free babysitting from someone you know and who has the experience of being a parent.

Paying for it

Various grants, credits and vouchers can be used to help offset the high costs of childcare. This section is not an exhaustive explanation of each system and of course is only accurate as at the time of print!

Nursery Education Grant

This grant enables your children to free part-time childcare from the term after their third birthday. The childcare provider, not the parent, claims the grant. Not all providers of childcare are eligible to claim it, so you should always check first. The grant covers up to five sessions per week of up to two-and-a-half hours per session. If your child attends sessions that are longer, often the case at daycare nurseries, then you will have to pay a top-up fee for the remaining time. Your childcare provider will make the application for the grant for children when they become eligible.

Childcare Voucher Schemes

This is a tax-free way of paying for your childcare, in which both your employer and your childcare provider need to participate. The vouchers are provided and administered by a third party. Voucher providers include:

- Accor Services   *www.childcarevouchers.co.uk*
- Busybees   *www.busybees.com*
- Childcare Choice   *www.childcarechoice.co.uk*
- Early Years vouchers Ltd *www.childcare-vouchers.net*
- Kiddivouchers   *www.kiddivouchers.com*

You will need to fill out a form, as will your care provider. You will then receive the vouchers on your usual payday instead of (or in addition to) your salary up to the allowed maximum, which at the time of print is £55.00 per week per working parent. Most of the schemes allow for you to receive 'e-vouchers' and for direct payments to be made to your care provider by the voucher provider. Otherwise you will receive paper vouchers that you hand over to your care provider and they then cash those in with the voucher provider.

The benefit to you is that you do not pay Income Tax or National Insurance on that £55.00 per week, making a potential saving of £1,196.00* per year with one parent claiming who is a higher rate taxpayer. A basic rate taxpayer will save up to £932.00* per year. The £55.00 limit applies to each individual and therefore if both parents are working and both their employers subscribe to a scheme, then between them they could receive vouchers for £110.00 per week. How much you can claim, and how much you will save will depend on your personal circumstances.

It is important to note that as the vouchers are shown as a reduction on your pay slip that it can affect entitlement to tax credits. For more guidance on how you may be affected go to *www.hmrc.gov.uk/menus/credits.htm*. Your employer saves the National Insurance on your childcare vouchers so if it doesn't currently offer them, it is worth your providing the details of the voucher scheme providers. It is worth noting that nannies and au pairs approved under the *Ofsted Childcare Register* or *Childcare Approval Scheme* can accept the vouchers as well as registered childcare providers, such as nurseries and childminders.

*from the Busybees website (www.busybeesvouchers.com) June 2007

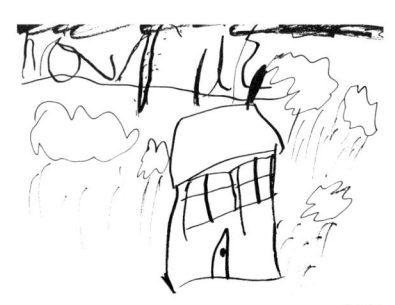

Childcare

BARROW HILLS SCHOOL

Roke Lane, Witley,
Godalming, Surrey, GU8 5NY
Tel: 01428 683639
E-mail: info@barrowhills.org.uk
www.barrowhills.org.uk
Registered Charity No. 1000190

Successful Catholic Day School for girls and boys aged 3 to 13
We welcome pupils from all denominations and support them within a Christian caring ethos

---

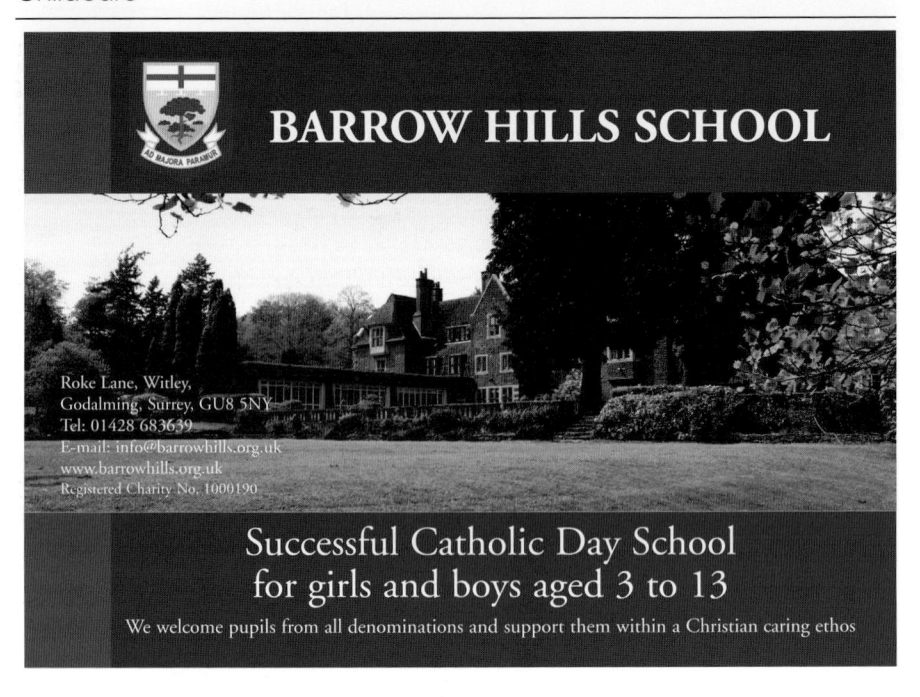

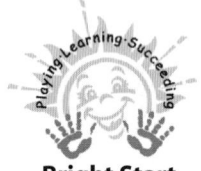

Bright Start Pre-School

A friendly, caring and community based Pre-School with over 30 years experience of quality care and education for 2½ to 4 year olds.

**A member of the Pre-School Learning Alliance.
OFSTED Inspected and Excellent OFSTED Report.**

The Pre-School is open on Monday, Tuesday, Thursday & Friday, from 9:15am to 12:15pm, at the United Reformed Church Hall, 83 Portsmouth Road, Guildford (opposite St. Nicholas' Infant School).

There is an outdoor play area and lots of (optional) opportunities for parental involvement.

For further information, or, for an appointment to view, please telephone Thea Arthur on:
01483 565298 during Pre-School hours.

DELANEY INTERNATIONAL

We have
AUSTRALIAN & ENGLISH
Nannies and Mother's Helps
plus
EUROPEAN Au Pairs
Call Marcia Delaney on
Guildford (01483) 894300
Fax: (01483) 894700
email: info@delaney-nannies.com
www.delaney-nannies.com

Bramble Cottage
Thorncombe Street
Bramley
Surrey GU5 0ND

Childcare

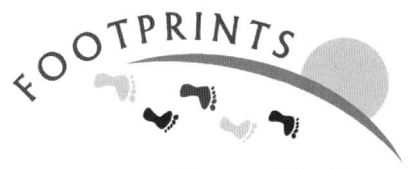

FOOTPRINTS
Montessori Day Nursery

For children aged 0-5 years

Owner managed

Purpose built giving space and light in all areas

A wonderful place to work and play

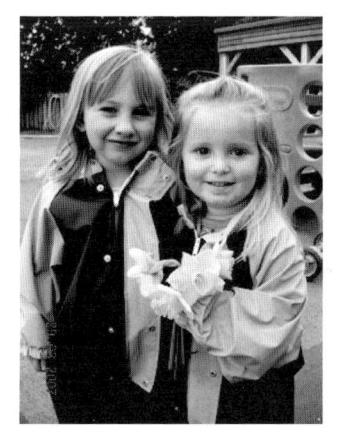

Resident cook provides nutritious meals

Offering care and education, following the Montessori philosophy and 'Every Child Matters'

Set in the midst of the Surrey countryside in beautifully converted barns offering children the opportunity to grow and develop at one with nature

Open 51 weeks of the year from 8am to 6pm Monday to Friday

Safe, homely and stimulating environment

Experienced, qualified and caring staff

Come and experience our atmosphere of peace and tranquillity, we will be happy to show you round our beautiful Nursery

Contact Sandra or Melanie on 01483 285591
A unique nursery in a unique setting

Childcare

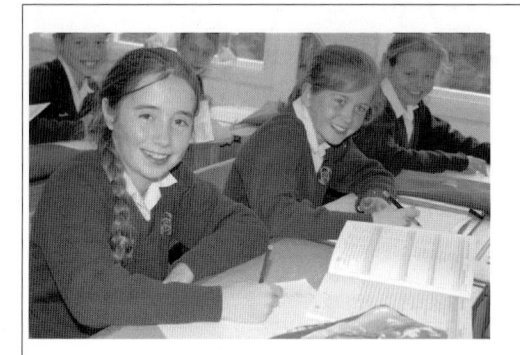

Excellent results
Superb facilities   Scholarships available

Giving your child a head start

registrar@sthilarysschool.com
www.sthilarysschool.com
Holloway Hill, Godalming
01483 - 416551

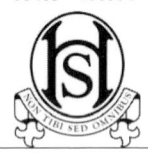

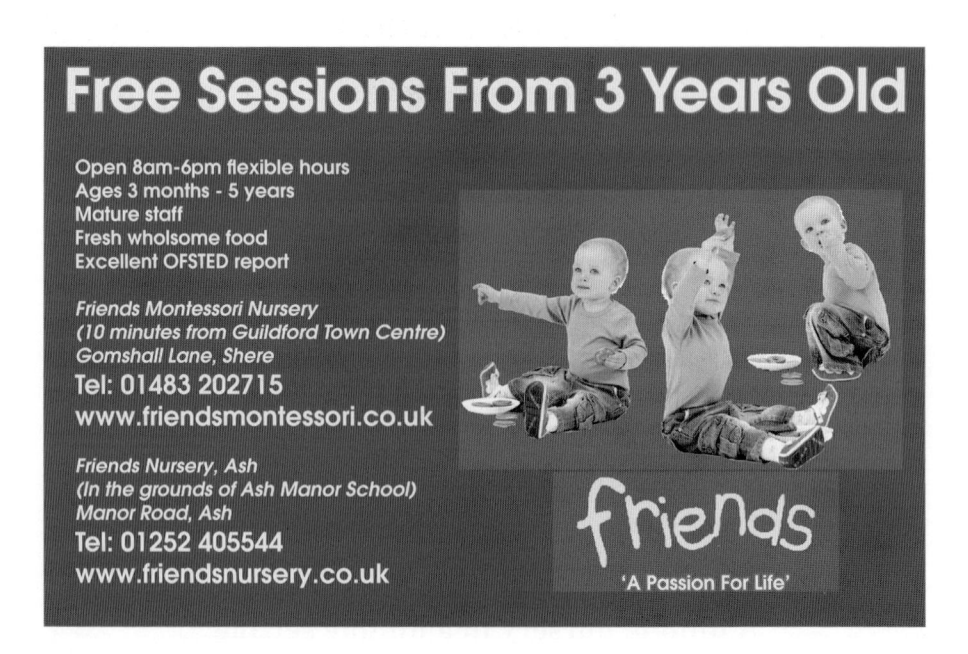

ST HILARY'S SCHOOL
IAPS Preparatory Day School
Boys 2½-7, Girls 2½-11

Free Sessions From 3 Years Old

Open 8am-6pm flexible hours
Ages 3 months - 5 years
Mature staff
Fresh wholsome food
Excellent OFSTED report

Friends Montessori Nursery
(10 minutes from Guildford Town Centre)
Gomshall Lane, Shere
Tel: 01483 202715
www.friendsmontessori.co.uk

Friends Nursery, Ash
(In the grounds of Ash Manor School)
Manor Road, Ash
Tel: 01252 405544
www.friendsnursery.co.uk

friends
'A Passion For Life'

Childcare

**DEUTSCHE SAMSTAGSSCHULE
WOKING/GUILDFORD**

German Saturday School
for bilingual children from 3 years onwards

At Pirbright Village Primary School
(term-times only) from 10am – 12pm

For more information please visit our website:
www.germanschool.co.uk
or call us on 07779 802 698 or 01483 487231

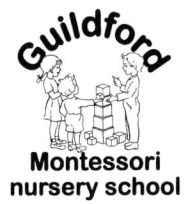

Guildford Montessori nursery school

Quality care and education

Open Monday – Friday
9.30 a.m. – 12.15 p.m.
Ages 2- 5 years

Free French, yoga, music sessions
Small group sizes
Outside play area
Optional lunch club

Tel: 0 780 730 90 25 / 01252 326458
surreymontessori@aol.com

St. Nicolas' C of E Infant School
Guildford's best kept educational secret

✓ Beautiful, peaceful location
✓ Strong community values
✓ Happy, confident children
✓ Nurturing and caring
✓ Excellent academic record
✓ Life-long love of learning

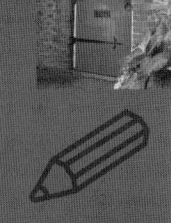

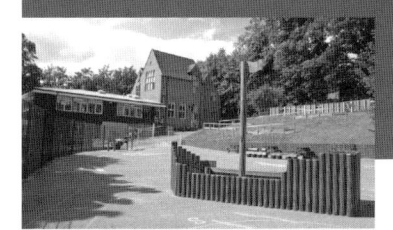

Portsmouth Road Guildford GU2 4YD
To find out more please call
01483 561639 or email

info@st-nicolas-guildford.surrey.sch.uk
www.st-nicolas-guildford.com

Pedestrian entrance via steps opposite the church on Portsmouth Road or via The Mount **Vehicle** entrance on Portsmouth Road next to Mount Pleasant

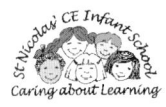

St Nicolas' CE Infant School — Caring about Learning

Acknowledgements

I would like to thank the following people for their help in producing this book:
- All the mums and dads who wrote reviews (and their children)
- The pupils (and teachers) of Onslow Infant School for their wonderfully poignant illustrations
- Claire Brown for initiating this new edition
- Debbie Beasley, typesetter and printing
- The chapter editors who collected and collated the initial reviews: Helen Ayscough, also treasurer; Kay Collins; Lynn Egan; Lise Faccinello; Kelley Friel; Jenny Kingston; Liz Robinson, also secretarial duties; Maggie Sherborne; Victoria Speirs, also marketing and sales; Dimitra Stamogiannou; Julie Stott, Katherine Thompson, also NCT head office liaison
- Also Tessa Davidson, committee secretary and advertising; Bally Ames, advertising, marketing and sales; Becky Kerby, proof reading and indexing; Renee Chow, Sandra May, Maja Pawinska Sims, Thora Thorsdottir and Cerys Byrne (NCT Head Office)
- Magnus Rew, Louise Wilson and Georgina Hayne, for providing me with a basis to develop on the original cover design
- Our advertisers, whose revenue made this publication possible. If you contact anyone you see advertised in the book, please let them know where you saw it.
- All the husbands and children of everyone involved. Special thanks from me to Chris, Charlotte and Louis, my brother, Leigh Apted, for his radio station *ISS Atlantis* on *live365.com* and my parents, Peter and Kathleen Apted, for their week-long stints at minding my children
- And finally, you the readers, who have kept that copy of the last edition of *Tots About Town* on your bedside tables, and have constantly encouraged me to give you an updated edition!

Please take this book, and use it to enrich the lives of you and your children. Enjoy, and be happy.

Emma Tappenden

Acknowledgements

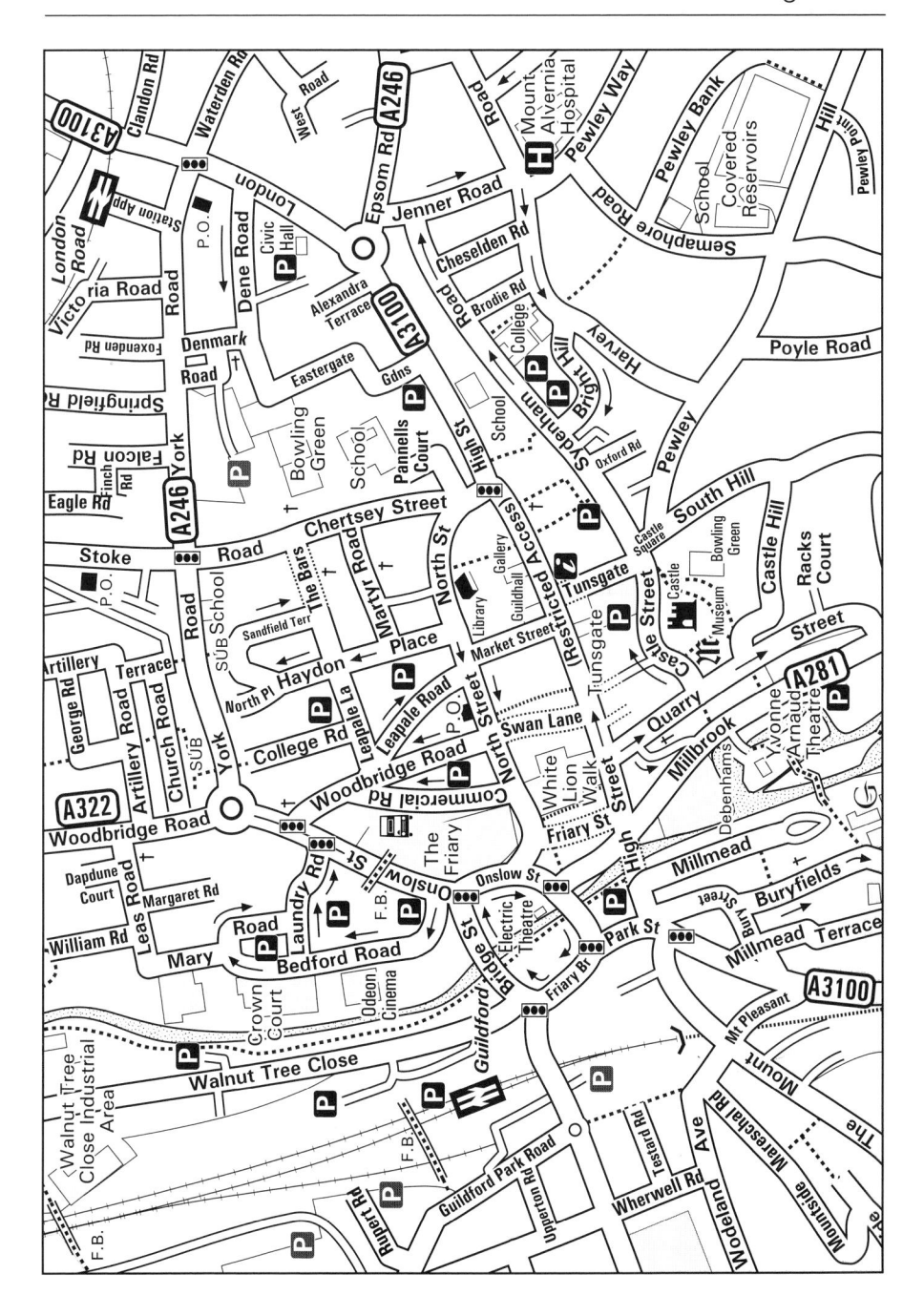

Acknowledgements

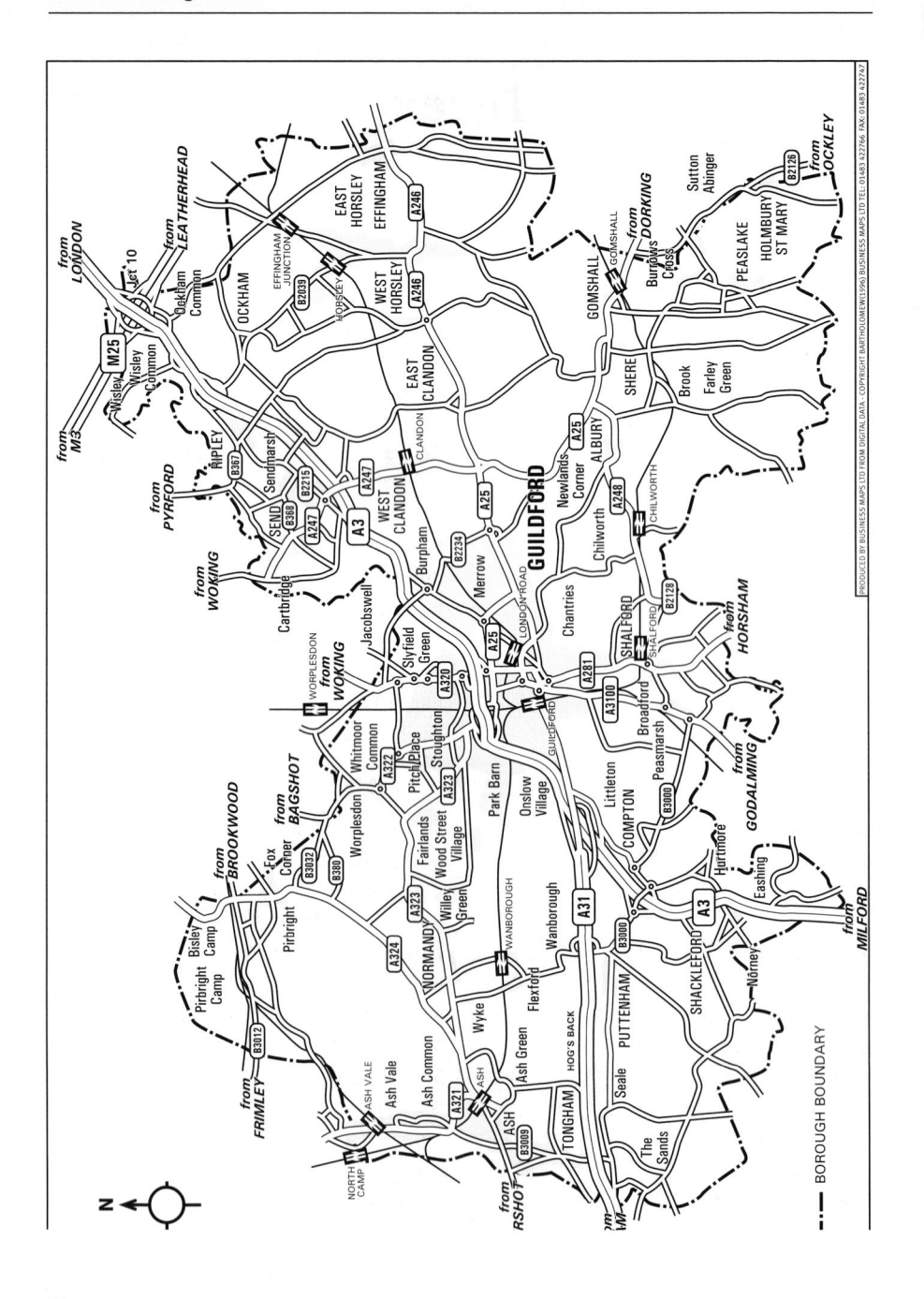

Index

06 Pottery Café, The 57-8
1 to 6 Gym Club 23
Abacus Baby and Party Hire 187
Abel & Cole 133-4
Abinger Hammer 77, 90, 107
Accessorize 122
aeroplanes 95, 97, 98, 103
Alice Holt Forest 86-8
Alice in Wonderland 77
Amberley Working Museum 92
animals *see* farms *and* zoos
antenatal classes 5, 9
ante/postnatal exercise 54-5, 60-4
Aquaschool 29-31
Aqua Pups 32
Aqua Tots 32
aquariums 71-4, 76, 80, 84
Argos 132
art activities 15, 21, 57-9, 63, 66, 80, 82, 92, 93, 96, 170
Ask 141
Aspace 134
Auberge 141, 157
au pairs 205
Babies 'R' Us *see* Toys 'R' Us
Baby Bargains of Ash 136
Baby Bounce and Rhyme 46, 167, 187
baby massage 54-5
babysitting 206
Baby Swimming 31-2
badminton 62

ballet *see* dance classes
Bar Centro 141
basketball 23, 41
Beale Park 71
Beano's 155
Beaulieu Abbey and Motor Museum 92-3
Bel and the Dragon 141-2
BHS 120
bird parks 71-3
Birdworld 71-2
Black Swan, The 156
Blooming Marvellous 125-6
Blubeckers Restaurants 109, 142
Bluebell Railway 98
bluebells 81, 82, 89
Blue Reef Aquarium 71
boat trips 80
Bocketts Farm 68, 105
Boden, Mini 134
Boogie Babies 55
Book People, The 134
bookshops 123, 128-32, 134
Boots 125, 139
bouncy castles 24, 38, 40, 42, 43, 45, 65, 66, 67, 98, 103, 168, 169, 171-2
bowling 23
Bracknell Leisure Centre 35
Brands Hatch Circuit 98-9
bras for breastfeeding 5, 125
Brasserie Chez Gérard 143
breast pumps 5

215

Index

breastfeeding support 5, 127, 133, 197-8
breastfeeding-friendly restaurants 139, 141, 149, 150, 151, 153, 154, 156
Brewers Fayre 156-7
bring and share meals 6, 8
Brooklands Museum 93, 99
Bump to 3 134
bumps and babes 6
Burpham Court Farm Park 69
bus information 115-8
Bushey Park 83
Café Rouge 142-3
Caffè Nero 150
Café Net 150-1
Café Revive 151-2
Café Zest 152
Campbell, Louise 197
car boot sales 137
Carluccio's Caffé 143
Carousel 128
catering equipment hire 174
Caterpillar Café 20, 64
changing facilities 16, 19, 33, 38, 39, 40, 42, 44, 45, 58, 72, 73, 74, 76, 79, 81, 82, 83, 84, 85, 86, 91, 93, 98, 99, 101, 102, 105, 120, 121, 122, 125, 127, 129, 130, 132, 138-9 *see also* Chapter 6: Eating Out
Chantry Wood 88
Chelsea Indoor Football Coaching 28, 65
Chessington World of Adventures 97
childcare 34, 199-211
childminders 202-3
Children's Centre *see* Guildford Children's Centre
chiropractors 193-4
Christmas events 75, 76, 82, 83, 85, 98, 104-6
Church, Sarah 55
churches 60, 64, 77, 88, 89, 103, 104, 105-6 *see also* parent and toddler groups
cinemas 51-4

circuit training 60-2
Citizens Advice Bureau 186-7
Clandon Park 74, 79-80, 116
Clandon Park Garden Centre 74
Claremont Landscape Garden 80, 116
Clarks 123-4, 128
clothes shops 120-3, 125, 126, 129, 133, 137-8
coffee mornings 6 *see also* parent and toddler groups
Compton Woods 89
Continental Café 152-3
Coral Reef 35
Cosmic Kids Club 22-3 *see also* Guildford Spectrum Leisure Complex
Costa Coffee 120, 153
counselling 197
craft activities *see* art activities
cranial osteopaths 194-5
Crazy Tots 38-9
crèche facilities 34-5, 60, 62, 63, 64, 99, 203-4
cycling 77, 85, 86-90, 95, 112
Da Gennaro 144
dance classes 55-7
Dapdune Wharf 80
daycare nurseries 200-1, 209
Debenhams 120, 133, 138, 144-5
deer 83, 85
Denbies Wine Estate 83
dentists 195-6
Diana, Princess of Wales' Memorial Playground 108
Disney Store 129
doctor's surgeries *see* GP surgeries
duck feeding 73, 76, 77-9, 80, 83, 97, 107, 109, 110, 111, 113, 114, 160, 189
Duckling Club 32-3
Dunk Your Bump 62
Early Learning Centre 120, 125, 129, 138
Easter events 81, 85, 98, 102
Electric Theatre, The 52, 53, 153

216

Index

Enchanted Wood 129, 131
Entertainer, The 129-30
entertainers 102, 174
equipment shopping 120, 125-8, 130, 135, 136, 137
equipment hire 5, 174, 187
Esporta Health and Fitness Club 34
exercise classes *see* ante/postnatal exercise
experience register 6, 7
Fairoaks Airport 99
farms 68-70, 71, 72, 74, 75, 97, 105
Farncombe Fun Zone 39, 167, 172
fetes 103
fireworks 104
Firing Earth 58
Fishers Farm Park 69
Fizzy Kids 39-40
football 25, 28-29, 41, 114
Formes 126
Forum Restaurant 156
Frensham Pond 90
Friary Centre 120, 121, 123-4, 126, 128. 129, 133, 138, 139, 153-4
Friday Street 90-1
Fruiti Boost Smoothie Bar 154
furniture 132-3, 134, 135, 137
Gap Kids 121
garden centres 74-7
Garden Room 154
gardens 79-86, 92-3, 108, 111
German school 211
Giraffe 145
Godalming School of Dance 55-6
Godstone Farm 70
GP surgeries 191-3
Great Little Trading Company 134-5
Grobag 134, 137
Guildford Book Festival 104
Guildford Borough Council 68, 106, 117, 166, 179, 184

Guildford Castle 83-4
Guildford Cathedral 89
Guildford Children's Centre 13, 14, 18, 64-5, 201
Guildford Comics and Games 130
Guildford House Gallery 93
Guildford Institute Restaurant 155
Guildford Lido 35-6
Guildford NCT 5-10, 30
Guildford Shakespeare Company 84
Guildford Spectrum Leisure Complex 7, 22, 23, 25, 27, 28, 30, 32-3, 36-7, 43-4, 46, 47, 60, 61, 62, 63, 64, 65, 116, 204
Guildford train station 99
Gunwharf Quays Outlet Village 100-1
gymnastics 23-7, 65-6
Gym Jams 40-1, 65, 168
Gymnastics Factory 23-4, 25, 65-6, 168, 169
Gympups 65
hairdressers 175-8
Hampton Court 83, 84
Hands of Clay 58-9
Harrison, Monique 54
Harvester restaurant 74
Haslemere Museum 94
Hatchlands Park 81
health visitors 192-3
Herons Swimming and Fitness Centre, The 34-5, 45, 63-4, 169
holiday activities 45, 52, 64-6, 68, 79, 80, 88, 92, 98, 100, 101
home birth 6
Horsham Pavilions in the Park 37
Horton Park Children's Farm 70
House of Fraser 117, 121, 152
ice skating 23, 29
Ice Pups 29
Ikea 132-3
INTECH Science and Discover Centre 94
internet shopping *see* online shopping

217

Index

Italia Conti Arts Centre 56
Jakes 41
Jan Harley Swim School 33-4
Jolly Farmer, The 92
JoJo Maman Bébé 126
Jo Shmo's 145
Kew Gardens 84, 117
Kiddicare 135
Kids Inc nursery 34
Kontinental Kids 121
Leatherhead & Dorking Gymnastics Club 24, 66
Leatherhead Leisure Centre 38-9
Legoland 97-8
libraries 5, 187-9
Guildford Library 46, 59-60, 66, 166-7, 186, 187-8
mobile library 66, 186, 188
NCT branch library 5, 129
toy library, Godalming 66, 172, 186, 188-9
lido *see* Guildford Lido
Little Angels *see* Rokers Little Angels
Little Green Frogs 46-7
Little Kickers 26, 28
Little Sparks 52, 53
Little Surrey Song Birds 46, 47
Little Treasures 185
Littletums 194
Loch Fyne 145-6
London Aquarium 117
London Eye 100, 117
Look Out Discovery Centre 94-5
Loseley Park 84-5
mail order shopping *see* online shopping
Manor Inn Beefeater 157
Marks and Spencer 121-2, 128, 139, 151-2
maternity wear 123, 125-8, 137-8
Mercedes-Benz World 93, 99
Mill, Elstead 157
Mill, Gomshall 142

Mill Studio, The 51
Millets 122
Mini IQ 128
model trains 103-4, 106
Monsoon 122
Moss, E. Pharmacy 128
Mothercare 127-8, 139
Mother Mentor, the 64
Mottisfont Abbey 81
Mucky pups 170
museums 80, 92-7
Music Box, The 47, 51
music groups 46-9, 50, 52, 53
Music with Mummy 47-8
nannies 204-5, 208
nappies 135, 179
nappy reps 181-5
National Childbirth Trust 3-10, 30, 33, 182, 184
NCT Nearly New Sales 7, 30, 137-8
NCT Swimming 7, 30, 33
National Trust 79-83, 90
Naturebotts 135
NCT *see* National Childbirth Trust
nearly new 7-8, 136, 137-8
Nell's Country Kitchen 155
Newland's Corner 91
Next 122-3
Notcutts Garden and Pet Centre 75
nurseries *see* daycare nurseries
Ocado 135-6
Odeon Guildford 52-4
Olivo Ristorante 146
online shopping 133-7 *see also* nappies
Onslow Arms, The 157
Onslow Village Arboretum 109-10
opticians 196-7
organic produce 133-4, 136
Organised Mum 127
paddling 36, 69, 71, 72, 77-78, 90, 111

218

Index

Painshill Park 85
parent & toddler groups 12-22
parks 79-80, 81, 83-6, 106-114
Parrot Inn, The 158
parties 39, 68, 70, 136, 167-74, 187
Patricia Ellis School of Dancing 56
Paultons Park 98, 105
Percy Arms, The 158
personal fitness training 62
photographers 178-9, 180
Pick 'n' Mix Playstore 44-5
Pizza Express 146-7
Pizza Hut 147
Planet Dance 57
play areas, outdoor 14, 18, 20, 37, 64-5, 68, 69, 70, 71, 72, 73, 74, 75, 77, 78, 80, 83, 84, 86-8, 94-5, 99, 100, 106-14, 188-9 *see also* pubs and bars
Polesden Lacey 81-2
Pool in the Park *see* Woking Leisure Centre
Portsmouth 100-1
postnatal groups 9 *see also* ante/postnatal exercise
Pottersline Nursery 75
pottery 57-9
Potty Paintbrush 59
powerpramming 58, 64
preschools 201-12, 208-211
Primark 123
public transport 73, 99, 101, 115-8
pubs and bars 91, 110, 156-161
quad biking 69
RAF Museum London 95
raft race 103
Rainbow Tots 41-2, 66, 170
Rajdoot Tandoori Restaurant 147
Ramster 85
Red Lion pub 110
reflexology 54-5
restaurants 101, 141-50 *see also* cafés *and*

pubs and bars
Richmond Park 85
Riverbank Café Bar 155
Riverford 136
rivers and canals 77, 78, 80, 81, 83, 109, 142, 144, 155, 156, 157, 159
Roald Dahl Museum and Story Centre 95-6
Rokers Little Angels 42, 116
Royal Surrey County Hospital 193, 196, 197
Runabout Indoor Soft Play Centre 42-3
Rushmoor Gym 24-5, 43, 66
Russell & Bromley 124
Ryder, Linda 56-7
schools 208-11
science discovery centres 94-5, 96
Science Museum 94, 96
Seahorse, The 160
seasonal events 69, 80, 82, 85, 98, 101-6
Seasons 137
second-hand shops *see* nearly new
Secretts Garden Centre 75
Sheepleas 91
shoe shops 123-5, 137-8
shops 119-39, 172-3, 174 *see also* nearly new, garden centres, parks *and* museums
signing 49-51
Sing a Song of Sixpence 48-9
Sing and Sign 49-50
singing classes *see* music groups
skating *see* ice skating
Socatots 28
soft play 18, 23, 24, 35, 37, 38-45, 65, 66, 68, 69, 70, 71 *see also* parties
Specky's Gympups 25, 65
Specky's Pirate Ship 23, 43-4
Spectrum *see* Guildford Spectrum Leisure Complex
sporting activities 22-38
Squires Garden Centre 76
Starbucks 112, 156

219

Index

Stars 123
Stephan Langton, The 91
Stoke Pub & Pizzeria 160
Stoke Park 101-2, 103-4, 111, 116
storytime 59-60
Strada 148
supermarket shopping 135-6
Surrey County Show 101-2
Sutherland Memorial Park 112-3, 116
swimming 7, 23, 29-37, 62, 63, 66, 69, 90
Swimming Academy, The 35
takeaways 161-5
tea rooms *see* cafés and bars
tennis 23, 65, 109, 111
TGI Friday's 148
theatres 51-52, 53
theme parks 97-8
Thomas the Tank Engine 72, 98, 100, 102
Three Horseshoes, The 158-9
Tickseed 136
Time to Sign 50
Tiny Talk 50-1
Toad Hall 44
toddler groups *see* parent and toddler groups
toilets 35, 38, 39, 40, 43, 44, 45, 69, 70, 73, 78, 81, 86, 88, 90, 91, 102, 105, 107, 108, 109, 112, 120, 121, 122, 125, 129, 130, 132, 133, 138-9
Tots Trampolining 27
Tourist Information Centre 167, 186, 189
toy shops 76, 123, 125, 128-32, 133, 134-5, 136, 137-8
Toys 'R' Us 130
tractor rides 68, 69, 70, 73
train rides 74, 83, 103-4
trains *see* vehicles *and* train rides
trampolining 23, 24, 25, 26, 27-8, 40, 43, 65, 66
Trotters 123, 124, 125, 178
Tumble Tots 25-6, 174

Underwater World 71-2
University of Surrey 27, 55
V&A Museum of Childhood 96
valley cushions 10
vehicles 80, 92-3, 95, 98-100, 103-4
Vertbaudet 137
Wagamama 148-9, 165
Waitrose 184, 186
walks 77, 78, 79-92, 94, 106, 107, 108, 109, 111, 158, 159, 160 *see also* gardens
Watercress Line 100, 102, 104, 117
Waterstones 130, 153
Weald & Downland Open Air Museum 97
Weyside, The 159
White Hart, The 159
White Horse, The 159-60
Whitmoor Common 91-2
WHSmith 132
Wildfowl and Wetlands Trust Arundel Wetland Centre 73
Willow Sanctuary 54
Windsor Great Park 85-6
Winkworth Arboretum 82-3
Wisley RHS Garden 86, 116
wizards 104
Wizzy World 44
Woking Gymnastics Club 26-7, 66
Woking Leisure Centre 44-5, 66
Woking Pool in the Park 33, 34, 37
Wooden It Be Lovely 132
Woolworths 133
Worplesdon Place 160-1
Wyevale Garden Centre 76-7
YMCA 156, 171
yoga 54-5
Yvonne Arnaud Theatre 51, 155
Zebedee's Music 48, 49
Zizzi 149-50
zoos 72-4